# ANTIMICROBIAL RESISTANCE - A GLOBAL THREAT

Edited by **Yashwant Kumar**

**Antimicrobial Resistance - A Global Threat**
http://dx.doi.org/10.5772/intechopen.73725
Edited by Yashwant Kumar

**Contributors**

Marina Spinu, Mihaela Niculae, Emoke Pall, Carmen Dana Sandru, Silvana Popescu, Christian Agyare, Vivian Etsiapa Boamah, Crystal Ngofi Zumbi, Frank Boateng Osei, Sonja Smole Možina, Vita Rozman, Bojana Bogovič Matijašić, Mariya Munir, Fateme Barancheshme, Funmilola Ayeni, Ayorinde Afolayan, Adewale Adetoye, Yenizey Merit Alvarez Cisneros, Edith Ponce-Alquicira, Yashwant Kumar



First published in London, United Kingdom, 2019 by IntechOpen
IntechOpen is the global imprint of INTECHOPEN LIMITED, registered in England and Wales, registration number: 11086078, The Shard, 25th floor, 32 London Bridge Street
London, SE19SG – United Kingdom
Printed in Croatia

British Library Cataloguing-in-Publication Data
A catalogue record for this book is available from the British Library

Additional hard copies can be obtained from orders@intechopen.com

Antimicrobial Resistance - A Global Threat, Edited by Yashwant Kumar
p. cm.
Print ISBN 978-1-78985-783-2
Online ISBN 978-1-78985-784-9
eBook (PDF) ISBN 978-1-83880-636-1

For EU product safety concerns:
IN TECH d.o.o., Prolaz Marije Krucifikse Kozulić 3, 51000 Rijeka, Croatia,
info@intechopen.com or visit our website at intechopen.com.

# Meet the editor

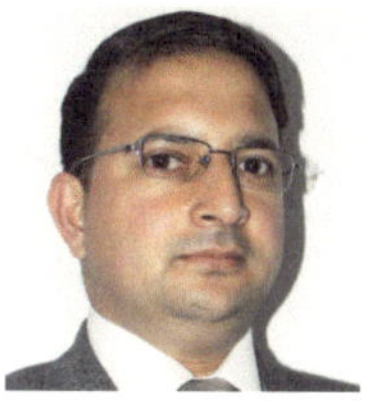

Dr. Yashwant Kumar is currently working as an officer in-charge of the National Salmonella and Escherichia Centre and Diagnostic Reagents Manufacturing Laboratory at the Central Research Institute, Kasauli (HP), India. He has more than 13 years of experience in epidemiology, surveillance, bacterial characterization, determination of antibiogram profiles, virulence factors, characterization of resistance markers, etc. He is also involved in academic programs and has supervised postgraduate and doctoral students during their research studies. Dr. Kumar has 27 publications in national and international peer-reviewed journals. He is also the editor of a book and other publications such as abstracts and a reviewer for a number of national and international journals. He has been trained in instrumental methods for drug analysis, advanced techniques in molecular biology and microbial technology, and biorisk management. He is a member of WHO-GFN (Global Foodborne Infections Network) and BIS for diagnostics, and he has also acted as an expert member for a project approved by DSIR.

# Contents

# Preface

Antimicrobial resistance (AMR) has emerged as the most serious global health concern. AMR hampers effective prevention and treatment of infections due to the ever-increasing range of bacteria that are becoming more powerful because of the development of novel resistance mechanisms against existing and newer antibiotics. Although AMR occurs naturally in bacteria, indiscriminate use of antibiotics in the human health sector and in livestock production is accelerating its development and spread to otherwise nonresistant bacteria through different modes. Different agencies such as the World Health Organization recognized AMR as a global threat and emphasized the need for an improved and coordinated global effort to control it.

An increasing number of infections, which were earlier easy to control, are now difficult to treat due to the development of resistance, further leading to increased medical costs, longer stays in hospital, and increased morbidity. Considering the prevailing scenario of antimicrobial resistance, urgent and sincere efforts are required right from the level of individuals to the level of policymakers to curb the resistance crisis. Moreover, there is a need to change antibiotic usage behavior, wherein the way to prescribe and use antibiotics should be looked into because unregulated usage of antibiotics is the most significant factor in the development of AMR.

To deal with this crisis, various aspects of AMR should be taken into consideration, including the study of prevailing antibiogram patterns among different bacteria from humans, animals, and the environment; development of newer classes of antibiotics to combat resistance mechanisms; detection of novel targets for antibiotics; reconsideration of conventionally used drugs showing re-emergence of susceptibility; and development as well as evaluation of alternative therapies.

This book contains seven chapters discussing different aspects of AMR. The first chapter is an introduction to the magnitude of the problem of antibiotic resistance, its causes, and mitigation strategies. The second chapter highlights the importance of antibiotic resistance in zoonotic bacteria. The problem of indiscriminate use of antibiotics in animal production and its role in the development of resistance is discussed in the third chapter. The fourth chapter discusses the problem of antibiotic resistance in lactic acid bacteria, whereas Chapter 5 highlights the development of resistance in wastewater treatment plants making them a significant source of environmental resistance. The sixth and seventh chapters describe alternative therapies: medicinal plants and beneficial microbes, respectively.

I put this book together with strong belief that it will provide information to all researchers working on the problem of AMR. The book will also help in understanding the seriousness of the problem and the necessity of framing strategies and policies to control the development and spread of antimicrobial resistance, in addition to the need for newer antibiotics and alternative therapies.

My heartfelt gratitude goes to Dr. A. K. Tahlan, Director, CRI, Kasauli, for his unwavering support throughout the book project. I would also like to thank my colleagues and subordinates for their unending motivation. Finally, my gratitude and love go to my family for their continuous inspiration and support.

**Dr. Yashwant Kumar**
National Salmonella and Escherichia Centre/Diagnostic Reagents Laboratory
Central Research Institute
Kasauli (HP), India

Chapter 1

# Introductory Chapter: Stepping into the Post-Antibiotic Era—Challenges and Solutions

Neelam Taneja, Shveta Sethi,
Ajay Kumar Tahlan and Yashwant Kumar

Additional information is available at the end of the chapter

http://dx.doi.org/10.5772/intechopen.84486

## 1. Antibiotics and antibiotic resistance in the pre-antibiotic era

Antibiotics are known to exist in the history of mankind since ancient times. They can be traced back to as early as 350–550 CE, when scientists found traces of tetracycline inhuman skeletal remains of ancient Sudanese Nuba [1]. This has led to the speculation that the diet of this population contained tetracycline. Even the red soils of Jordon which have been used since time immemorial to treat wounds have been shown to contain *Actinomycete* bacteria which produced actinomycin [2]. Antimicrobial activity is also present in many of the herbs used in traditional Indian Ayurvedic and Chinese medicines.

Antibiotics have saved countless lives, and at one point of time, we imagined that infectious diseases were conquered. Most of the advances of modern medicine including state of art surgeries and management of neutropenic, transplant and cancer patients are based on the use of effective broad-spectrum antibiotics. Thanks to the way we have handled these precious resources for treatment of variety of infectious diseases. However, we found to our dismay subsequently that we are stepping into the post-antibiotic era.

Antibiotic resistance genes have been present in nature long before the modern antibiotic era began. Some of the serine and metallo-beta-lactamases originated more than 2 million years ago [3]. It seems prudent to assume that the ancient bacteria had defence mechanisms (such as antibiotic altering enzymes or efflux pumps) to protect themselves from high antibiotic concentrations. Hence, the biosynthetic gene cluster that makes the "antibiotic" must also contain genes which confer "resistance" to these antibiotics, and many aspects of the resistome (collection of all AMR genes in a specific bacteria or ecological niche) might have developed much before these antibiotics became prevalent in clinical practice.

## 2. Modern antibiotic era

Modern antibiotic era began in 1904–1910 with Paul Ehrlich and Alexander Fleming [4, 5]. Initially, it was limited to the discovery of chemicals like inorganic mercury salts and organo-arsenic compounds to treat syphilis. It was Paul Ehrlich who introduced the systemic screening approach that is the cornerstone of modern drug research trials [4]. Paul Ehrlich and his team synthesised hundreds of organo-arsenic derivatives of a very toxic drug Atoxyl and tested them in rabbits infected with syphilis. This approach led to the discovery of Salvarsan and later to a sulfa drug (Prontosil). The serendipitous discovery of penicillin by Alexander Fleming in 1928 changed the history of infectious diseases [5]. It was Florey and Chain who led the pathway for purification of penicillin and later to its mass production [6]. Interestingly enough, Fleming was the one who sounded the warning bells regarding the development of resistance to the penicillin, if not used properly. So, in a nutshell, discovery of the first three antimicrobials, Salvarsan, Prontosil and penicillin paved the pathway for the discovery of newer antibiotics in future.

The golden era of discovery of newer antibiotics continued and lasted till 1970s when most of the major classes like tetracyclines, methicillin, gentamicin, etc. were discovered [7]. This was followed by apparent absence of newer drug discovery with occasional antibiotic making an appearance here and there. Simultaneously, we made each newly discovered antibiotic ineffective after its launch by extensive use and misuse for trivial illnesses. The prime example of this is the fluoroquinolone, ciprofloxacin [8]. It was one of the most active, broad-spectrum antibiotics which had minimum side effects and a very good bioavailability upon oral use and soon became a drug of choice for many infections. Its extensive usage for gastroenteritis and respiratory infections, which were mostly viral in origin, led to the development of high level of resistance especially in developing countries.

## 3. Antibiotic resistance: origin and current status

The first concern regarding antimicrobial resistance appeared with the observation of penicillin resistant *Staphylococcus* in 1940 [7]. Initial few observations suggested that bacteria could destroy the drug by enzymatic degradation. Shortly thereafter, penicillin resistance became a substantial clinical problem. The first case of methicillin-resistant *Staphylococcus aureus* (MRSA) was identified in the United Kingdom in 1962 and in the United States in 1968 [9, 10]. In reality, this is true for many other pathogenic bacteria, including the *Enterobacteriaceae*, which have become resistant not only to the original penicillin but also to semisynthetic penicillins, cephalosporins and newer carbapenems [11]. Details about the development of the resistance in different classes of antibiotics are shown in the timeline (**Figure 1**) [7]. Antimicrobial resistance often occurs through various mechanisms such as inhibition of cell wall synthesis, nucleic acid synthesis, ribosome function, protein synthesis, folate metabolism and cell membrane function. The target can be (i) modified, as in the case of acetylation of aminoglycosides, (ii) destroyed (as the β-lactam antibiotics by the

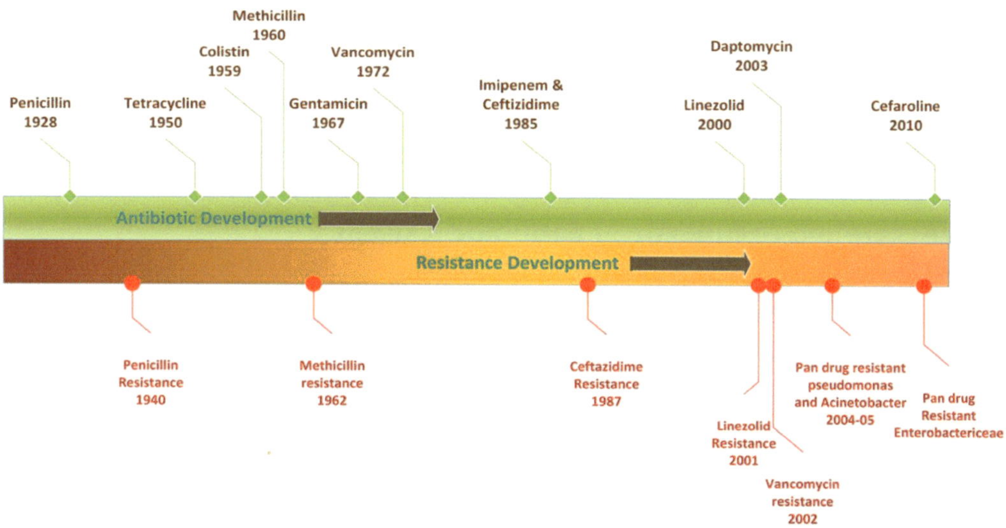


**Figure 1.** Timeline showing antibiotic development and antimicrobial resistance.

action of β-lactamases) and (iii) pumped out from the cell as in efflux pump mechanisms of resistance [12].

Unfortunately, true burden of antimicrobial resistance (AMR) remains unknown. There are many hindrances in estimating the burden of AMR. Incongruent data is available from public and private sectors; data are often not collected properly and contain little information of patient follow up. These problems are intensified in low- and middle-socioeconomic countries due to problems of inadequate surveillance, poor laboratory infrastructure and limited access to the crucial antimicrobials. According to a study from Vietnam and Thailand, prevalence of stool carriage of extended-spectrum beta-lactamase (ESBL)-producing *Escherichia coli* was 51.0 and 69.3%, respectively [13]. There is also an increasing prevalence of MDR Gram-positive bacteria. Another study in Thailand and Indonesia showed that prevalence of MRSA carriage is around 8% in admitted patients [14, 15]. Similar or worse situation exists in other Asian countries including China, Pakistan, Bangladesh and India. Antimicrobial resistance is a global issue. Resistance genes spread throughout the world as recent database lists the existence of more than 20,000 potential resistance genes (r genes) of nearly 400 different types, predicted from available sequences [16]. It is difficult to estimate the exact AMR burden due to the lack of comprehensive and uniform data. Gram-negative bacteria possessing the capabilities of producing extended-spectrum beta-lactamases (ESBL), AmpC beta-lactamases and carbapenemases have emerged as a therapeutic challenge for medical fraternity [17]. *Enterococcus faecium, Staphylococcus aureus, Klebsiella pneumoniae, Acinetobacter baumannii, Pseudomonas aeruginosa*, and *Enterobacter* species have been classified into a group known as "ESKAPE" due to their ability to escape the action of antimicrobials [18]. Multiple mechanisms of antimicrobial resistance have been acquired by carbapenem-resistant *Enterobacteriaceae* (CRE), *P. aeruginosa* and *A. Baumannii* resulting in enhanced morbidity and mortality [19–23]. In the 1990s, emergence of ESBLs among different microorganisms on global level led to widespread and increased use of carbapenems giving rise to emergence of pandemic CRE [24]. The Centers for Disease Control and Prevention has categorised CRE as *urgent* and ESBL-producing Gram-negative bacteria as *serious* antibiotic threats in the USA [10].

## 4. The scare and complexity of antibiotic resistance

The scale, to which antibiotic resistance has become a challenge in the treatment of the modern medicine, is scary to say the least. Every year, around 25,000 patients die of the infection with multidrug-resistant bacteria alone in the European Union [25]. In the United States alone, nearly 90,000 people die of hospital-acquired infections [26]. According to Jim O'Neill, >700,000 people die across the globe every year due to infections caused by multidrug-resistant organisms [27]. In this study, it was predicted that by 2050, more than 10 million people will die because of multidrug-resistant bugs. Huge economic losses are also expected, leading to reduction of 2–3.5% in GDP; livestock production will fall by 3–8%, costing the world up to $100 trillion [27]. Developing countries in Africa and South Asia will be the worst affected.

AMR is not only a problem of human medicine but also an ecological problem. Microbes have proved not only smarter than humans in developing new arsenal but also have armies in the form of biofilms. It looks like humans may be losing the arms race to bacteria, and the advent of the post-antibiotic era is imminent.

## 5. Causes of the antibiotic resistance crisis

### 5.1. Overuse

Antibiotic consumption is the single most important risk factor for emergence and spread of resistant bacterial strains. In many countries including India, antibiotics are easily available over the counter even without a prescription [28]. Moreover, antibiotics are plentiful and cheap also. This non-prescription use of drugs varies from 19 to 90% in various countries outside the United States and Europe, which is a matter of serious concern [29]. The problem has been compounded by the online purchase of these products, which further facilitate the self-medication. Some surveys reported that patients often do not know that they were prescribed an antimicrobial and the true proportion of patients using antimicrobials is probably higher than the reported [30, 31]. On the other hand, there are instances where patients demand antibiotics from their clinicians.

### 5.2. Inappropriate prescriptions

Incorrectly prescribed antibiotics contribute majorly to the burden of resistant bacteria. Several studies have observed that indication, choice of the antibiotics and duration of

http://dx.doi.org/10.5772/intechopen.84486

treatment are incorrect in almost 30–50% of cases [32, 33]. Extensive usage occurs in ICUs and high-dependency units, and there too approximately, 30–60% of the usage is unnecessary or incorrect [33]. Studies from pharmacies of Vietnam show that 90% of antimicrobials are sold without a proper prescription [34]. Upper respiratory tract infections (URTI) are good example, for which antimicrobial are commonly prescribed over the counter. This illustrates the overuse of antimicrobials for a condition that is often self-limiting and generally of viral aetiology. Suboptimal doses of any antibiotic further promote the genetic alterations as well as mutagenesis in the bacteria which lead to the development of multi-drug resistance in them.

### 5.3. Extensive use in livestock sector

Antibiotics are widely used as growth promoters and to prevent infections in the livestock sector. In the United States alone, an estimated 80% of the sold antibiotics are used in farm animals [7]. In 2010, India was one of the world's largest consumers of antibiotics in the veterinary sector [35]. The resistant bacteria reach the consumers through food animal products, mainly meat. These bacteria constitute large pools of AMR genes that can be transferred to humans and pathogenic bacteria by natural horizontal gene transfer mechanisms. These bacteria, although some may only be transient and do not colonise the intestinal tract, reside long enough to interact with the host microbiota and may possibly acquire or release genes. They can also act as opportunistic pathogens in susceptible hosts and probably play a key role in the evolution and dissemination of AMR. The use of antibiotics in food not only leads to the emergence and spread of resistant bacteria but also can be hazardous to many types of nontargeted environmental microorganisms. High concentrations of therapeutic antibiotics tend to be lethal to most bacterial strains leaving little opportunity for selection of subpopulations that have low or intermediate resistant traits. On the other hand, low levels of antibiotics in environment like soil, water and sewage become grounds for the selection of resistant microorganisms leading to the development of resistant gene pool or resistome [7, 12].

### 5.4. Availability of few new antibiotics

Investment in antibiotic development research is no longer considered as an economically wise decision for pharmaceutical companies [36]. According to a study conducted in London, it was calculated that the net present value (NPV) of new antibiotics is only about $50 million, compared to approximately $1 billion for a drug used to treat a neuromuscular disease [37].

Other reasons include low cost of antibiotics, regulatory barriers and tendency to save the new drug for serious infections. In spite of global warnings issued by many agencies, very few new drug discoveries fail to keep pace with worsening resistance scenario. As declared by the CDC in 2013, the human race is moving into a new era of infectious disease: the post-antibiotic period [38]. Here are few examples of the MDR organisms which are considered a substantial threat to the humankind. They have been divided as "urgent," "serious" or "concerning" by CDC [24, 39] (**Figure 2**).

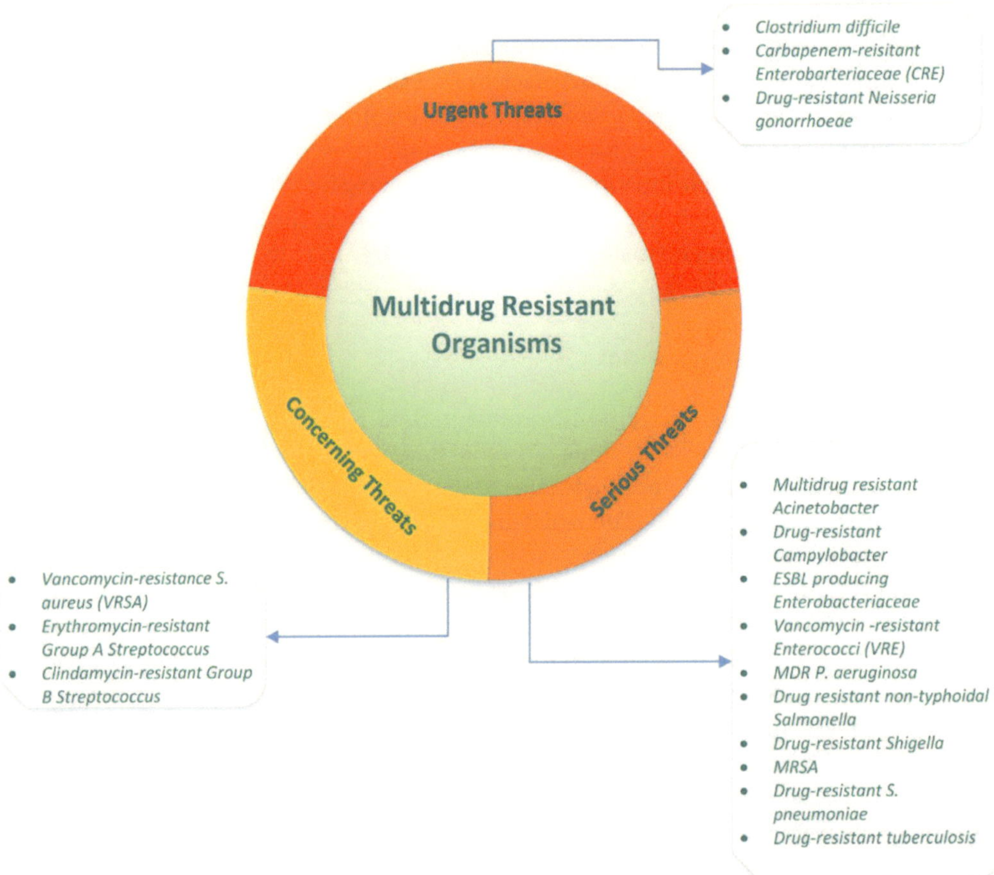


**Figure 2.** Urgent, concerning and serious threats with respect to development of antimicrobial resistance.

## 6. Solutions: do we have any?

There is an urgent need to strategize to save the existing antimicrobials. We can perform that by following means to improve the existing ones, discover novel antibiotics, dig up the old so-called toxic compounds, scale up antibiotic stewardship, use inter-sectorial multidisciplinary approaches, educate the public and clinician's alike and reduce the antibiotics in livestock and agriculture to name a few [12].

### 6.1. New targets/approaches

Soil and marine environments appear to be rich ecological niches to discover new agents and so do the plants and animals. Co-trimoxazole was a perfect example of targeting two enzymes in a metabolic pathway producing synergism. Compounds can be synthesised artificially to target more than one mechanism. There is important role of whole genome sequencing and metagenomics to find the new targets.

We hope that novel hitherto unknown mechanisms of antibiotic resistance will be revealed which can be exploited to find new targets. The drugs targeting anti-virulence mechanisms are an attractive strategy and have shown some promising results. Other interesting approach may be to target/alter untapped metabolic pathways like fatty acid synthesis, proton motive force, quorum sensing, signal transduction, efflux pumps, etc. [12]. Many of such compounds are currently in experimental stages.

### 6.2. Repurposing of compounds

Some of the compounds are already approved by FDA for treatment of metabolic disorders and cancers also have antimicrobial properties and can be repurposed, e.g., the compound BPH-652 that inhibits squalene synthase involved in cholesterol biosynthesis and also inhibits dehydrosqualene synthase involved in virulence in *Staphylococcus aureus*, hence a good candidate for Methicillin-resistant *Staphylococcus aureus* (MRSA) [12].

### 6.3. Considering conventional drugs

The drugs used in the past, which have been revived and now are used to treat the infections caused by Gram-negative bacteria, include colistin, fosfomycin, temocillin and rifampicin [17].

### 6.4. Combination therapy

Finding a suitable antimicrobial treatment option for some of the highly drug-resistant bacteria can be really daunting, and many times, clinicians resort to using combinations without data pertaining to their efficacy. The main drugs in these combinations are polymyxins and tigecycline; however, additional drugs comprise carbapenems, tigecycline, fosfomycin, aminoglycosides, and rifampicin [17] where data on randomised control trials of these drugs is also lacking. The factors which need to be taken into account before an appropriate combination is used includes the targeted organism and its susceptibility profile, co-morbidities present in the patient and the site of the infection. More studies including pharmacokinetic and pharmacodynamics studies are required to find the ideal combinations [40].

### 6.5. Phage therapy

Phages have the advantage of high specificity for their hosts without any notable adverse effects. They were historically in use in Europe for treatment of bacterial infections such as skin/wound infections, urinary tract infections, ear infections and even osteomyelitis [41]. New interest has been generated in phage therapy, and it may turn out to be a useful adjunct to antibiotics. Coupling antibiotics with phages or inhibitors of enzymes appears to be an attractive strategy which may succeed in many cases [41].

## 7. Prevention of further spread of AMR

The extent to which AMR has spread is due to the selective pressure provided by extensive antibiotic consumption and usage. Strategies to curtail the human use of antibiotic include antibiotic stewardship, public awareness to avoid self-medication, use of antibiotics in therapeutic doses and for appropriate length of time and education and counselling to patients not to pressurise the clinician into prescribing antibiotics for trivial illnesses. Development of new rapid diagnostic point of care tests will inform the clinician not to use antibiotics in the viral infections.

### 7.1. Regulation in human as well livestock sector

Though a sticky and complex issue, regulation of unprescribed antibiotics is essential especially in developing countries. There should be the rule of "prescription-only medicines" similar to various international guidelines [42]. In the veterinary and agriculture set-up, antibiotic usage is linked to economic gains. Scandinavian countries set up a good example to follow by not using antibiotics as growth promoters, and they do have the least AMR issues [43].

### 7.2. Antibiotic stewardship

Antimicrobial stewardship refers to "The optimal selection, dosage, and duration of antimicrobial treatment that results in the best clinical outcome for the treatment or prevention of infection, with minimal toxicity to the patient and minimal impact on subsequent resistance" [44]. Hence, antimicrobial stewardship basically aims at helping each patient receive the appropriate treatment without adverse effects of antibiotic use. These programmes are beneficial in reducing treatment failures, decreasing health-care associated infections and also reducing antibiotic resistance while proving economically beneficial to the hospital.

### 7.3. Connecting human, animal and environmental health: One Health Approach

In 2003, in an interview, a journalist used the word "One Health" by saying that "Human or livestock or wildlife health can't be discussed in isolation anymore-there is just one health" [45]. Since then "One Health" concept has gained more recognition in the public health and animal health communities. "One Health" is a collaborative approach among various sectors and disciplines to achieve optimal health outcomes emphasising the relation between humans, animals, plants and environment shared by them [46]. This is the need of the hour because many diseases are zoonotic in nature, and microbes harbouring drug-resistant genes have no barriers. Now the WHO and CDC have also adopted this approach.

## 8. Conclusions

The AMR is marching globally and threatens to undo the extraordinary advancements achieved in human medicine. Coordinated efforts are required across the globe to manage this great crisis. It is time we learn from our mistakes and gather our act together to outsmart the bacteria. All said and done, microbes do have an evolutionary advantage of nearly 4 billion years and have learnt to survive the onslaught of antibiotics. We can learn from them by using the sophisticated molecular approaches we have. Antimicrobial resistance is not only a human health problem but is an ecological challenge as well. It is up to the human race to take up this challenge and save the world from this menace.

## Author details

Neelam Taneja[1], Shveta Sethi[1], Ajay Kumar Tahlan[2] and Yashwant Kumar[2]

*Address all correspondence to: yasht26@yahoo.co.in

1 Postgraduate Institute of Medical Education and Research, Chandigarh, India

2 Central Research Institute, Kasauli, Himachal Pradesh, India

## References

[1] Nelson ML, Dinardo A, Hochberg J, Armelagos GJ. Brief communication: Mass spectroscopic characterization of tetracycline in the skeletal remains of an ancient population from Sudanese Nubia 350-550 CE. American Journal of Physical Anthropology. 2010;**143**:151-154

[2] Sobell HM. Actinomycin and DNA transcription. Proceedings of the National Academy of Sciences of the United States of America. 1985;**82**:5328-5331

[3] Garau G, Di Guilmi AM, Hall BG. Structure-based phylogeny of the metallo-beta-lactamases. Antimicrobial Agents and Chemotherapy. 2005;**49**:2778-2784

[4] Ehrlich P, Hata S. Die Experimentelle Chemotherapie der Spirilosen. Berlin: Julius Springer; 1910

[5] Fleming A. On antibacterial action of culture of Penicillium, with special reference to their use in isolation of *B. influenzae*. British Journal of Experimental Pathology. 1929;**10**:226-236

[6] Chain E, Florey HW, Gardner AD, Heatley NG, Jennings MA, Orr-Ewing J, et al. The classic: Penicillin as a chemotherapeutic agent. Clinical Orthopaedics and Related Research. 2005;**439**:23-26

[7] Ventola CL. The antibiotic resistance crisis part 1: Causes and threats. P&T. 2015;**40**:277-283

[8] Fasugba O, Gardner A, Mitchell BG, Mnatzaganian G. Ciprofloxacin resistance in community- and hospital-acquired *Escherichia coli* urinary tract infections: A systematic review and meta-analysis of observational studies. BMC Infectious Diseases. 2015;**15**:1-16

[9] Sengupta S, Chattopadhyay MK, Grossart HP. The multifaceted roles of antibiotics and antibiotic resistance in nature. Frontiers in Microbiology. 2013;**4**:47

[10] Center for Disease Control and Prevention. Office of Infectious Disease. Antibiotic resistance threats in the United States. 2013. Available from: http://www.cdc.gov/drugresistance/threat-report-2013

[11] Kumarasamy KK, Toleman MA, Walsh TR, Bagaria J, Butt F, Balakrishnan R, et al. Emergence of a new antibiotic resistance mechanism in India, Pakistan, and the UK: A molecular, biological, and epidemiological study. Lancet Infectious Diseases. 2010;**10**:597-602

[12] Aminov RI. A brief history of the antibiotic era: Lessons learned and challenges for the future. Frontiers in Microbiology. 2010;**1**:1-7

[13] Nakayama T, Ueda S, Huong BTM, Tuyen LD, Komalamisra C, Kusolsuk T, et al. Wide dissemination of extended-spectrum beta-lactamase-producing *Escherichia coli* in community residents in the Indochinese Peninsula. Infection and Drug Resistance. 2015;**8**:1-5

[14] Bunnueang N, Kongpheng S, Yadrak P, Rattanachuay P, Khianngam S, Sukhumungoon P. Methicillin-resistant *Staphylococcus aureus*: 1-year collection and characterization from patients in two tertiary hospitals, Southern Thailand. Southeast Asian Journal of Tropical Medicine and Public Health. 2016;**47**:234-244

[15] Kuntaman K, Hadi U, Setiawan F, Koendori EB, Rusli M, Santosaningsih D, et al. Prevalence of methicillin resistant *Staphylococcus aureus* from nose and throat of patients on admission to medical wards of Dr. Soetomo Hospital, Surabaya,Indonesia. The Southeast Asian Journal of Tropical Medicine and Public Health. 2016;**47**:66-70

[16] Davies J, Davies D. Origins and evolution of antibiotic resistance. Microbiology and Molecular Biology Reviews. 2010;**74**:417-433

[17] Taneja N, Kaur H. Insights into newer antimicrobial agents against gram-negative bacteria. Microbiology Insights. 2016;**9**:9-19

[18] Boucher HW, Talbot GH, Bradley JS, Edwards JE, Gilbert D, Rice LB, et al. Bad bugs, no drugs: No ESKAPE! An update from the Infectious Diseases Society of America. Clinical Infectious Diseases. 2009;**48**:1-12

[19] Tzouvelekis LS, Markogiannakis A, Psichogiou M, Tassios PT, Daikos GL. Carbapenemases in *Klebsiella pneumoniae* and other *Enterobacteriaceae*: An evolving crisis of global dimensions. Clinical Microbiology Reviews. 2012;**25**:682-707

[20] Daikos GL, Petrikkos P, Psichogiou M, Kosmidis C, Vryonis E, Skouteliet A, et al. Prospective observational study of the impact of VIM-1 metallo-beta-lactamase on the outcome of patients with *Klebsiella pneumoniae* bloodstream infections. Antimicrobial Agents and Chemotherapy. 2009;**53**:1868-1873

[21] Giamarellou H, Poulakou G. Multidrug-resistant Gram-negative infections: What are the treatment options? Drugs. 2009;**69**:1879-1901

[22] Marchaim D, Chopra T, Pogue JM, Perez F, Hujer AM, Rudin S, et al. Outbreak of colistin-resistant, carbapenem-resistant *Klebsiella pneumoniae* in metropolitan detroit, Michigan. Antimicrobial Agents and Chemotherapy. 2011;**55**:593-599

[23] Papp-Wallace KM, Endimiani A, Taracila MA, Bonomo RA. Carbapenems: Past, present, and future. Antimicrobial Agents and Chemotherapy. 2011;**55**:4943-4960

[24] Logan LK, Weinstein RA. The epidemiology of carbapenem-resistant Enterobacteriaceae: The impact and evolution of a global menace. The Journal of Infectious Disease. 2017; **215**(suppl 1):S28-S36

[25] Cotinat MC, Lacoste J, Buisson CB, Jarlier V, Coignard B, Vaux S. Estimating the morbidity and mortality associated with infections due to multidrug-resistant bacteria (MDRB), France, 2012. Antimicrobial Resistance and Infection Control. 2016;**5**:1-11

[26] Stone PW. Economic burden of healthcare-associated infections: An American perspective. Expert Review of Pharmacoeconomics & Outcomes Research. 2009;**9**:417-422

[27] O'Neill J; on behalf of the Review on Antimicrobial Resistance. Tackling Drug-Resistant Infections Globally: Final Report and Recommendations. 2016. https://amr-review.org/sites/default/files/160525_Final%20paper_with%20cover.pdf

[28] Panda A, Pradhan S, Kshatri JS. Predictors of over-the-counter medication: A cross-sectional Indian study. Perspectives in Clinical Research. 2017;**8**:79-84

[29] Editorial. The antibiotic alarm. Nature. 2013;**495**:141

[30] Alliance for the Prudent Use of Antibiotics. Executive summary: Select findings, conclusions, and policy recommendations. Clinical Infectious Diseases. 2005;**41**(suppl 4):224-227

[31] Morgan DJ, Okeke IN, Laxminarayan R, Perencevich EN, Weisenberg S. Non-prescription antimicrobial use worldwide: A systematic review. The Lancet Infectious Diseases. 2011; **11**:692-701

[32] Smieszek T, Pouwels KB, Dolk FCK, Smith DRM, Hopkins S, Sharland M, et al. Potential for reducing inappropriate antibiotic prescribing in English primary care. Journal of Antimicrobial Chemotherapy. 2018;**73**:ii36-ii43

[33] Luyt CE, Brechot N, Trouillet JL, Chastre J. Antibiotic stewardship in the intensive care unit. Critical Care. 2014;**18**:480

[34] Nga DTT, Chuc NTK, Hoa NP, Hoa NQ, Nguyen NTT, Loan HT, et al. Antibiotic sales in rural and urban pharmacies in northern Vietnam: An observational study. BMC Pharmacology & Toxicology. 2014;**15**:6

[35] Boeckel V, Brower TP, Gilbert C, Grenfell M, Levin BT, Robinson S, et al. Global trends in antimicrobial use in food animals. Proceedings of the National Academy of Sciences. 2015;**112**:5649-5654. DOI: 10.1073/pnas.1503141112

[36] Piddock LJ. The crisis of no new antibiotics—What is the way forward? Lancet Infectious Diseases. 2012;**12**:249-253

[37] Bartlett JG, Gilbert DN, Spellberg B. Seven ways to preserve the miracle of antibiotics. Clinical Infectious Diseases. 2013;**56**:1445-1450

[38] Michael CA, Dominey-Howes D, Labbate M. The antibiotic resistance crisis: Causes, consequences, and management. Frontiers in Public Health. 2014;**2**:145

[39] Rossolini GM, Arena F, Pecile P, Pollini S. Update on the antibiotic resistance crisis. Current Opinion in Pharmacology. 2014;**18**:56-60

[40] Poudyal A, Yu HH, Matthaiou DK. Colistin and doripenem combinations demonstrate synergy and suppression of resistance against *Acinetobacter baumannii* at multiple inocula in an in vitro PK/PD Model. In: 21st European Congress of Clinical Microbiology And Infectious Diseases (ECCMID); Milan. 2011

[41] Viertel TM, Ritter K, Horz HP. Viruses versus bacteria-novel approaches to phage therapy as a tool against multidrug-resistant pathogens. Journal of Antimicrobial Chemotherapy. 2014;**69**:2326-2336

[42] Davies SC. Reducing inappropriate prescribing of antibiotics in English primary care: Evidence and outlook. Journal of Antimicrobial Chemotherapy. 2018;**73**:833-834

[43] Bengtsson B, Wierup M. Antimicrobial resistance in Scandinavia after ban of antimicrobial growth promoters. Animal Biotechnology. 2006;**17**:147-156

[44] Gerding DN. The search for good antimicrobial stewardship. Joint Commission Journal on Quality Improvement. 2001;**27**:403-404

[45] Weiss R. Africa's Apes Are Imperiled, Researchers Warn. The Washington Post. Apr. 7, 2003

[46] Available from: https://www.cdc.gov/onehealth/index.html

Chapter 2

# Antimicrobial Resistance of Common Zoonotic Bacteria in the Food Chain: An Emerging Threat

Vita Rozman, Bojana Bogovič Matijašić and
Sonja Smole Možina

Additional information is available at the end of the chapter

http://dx.doi.org/10.5772/intechopen.80782

**Abstract**

Antimicrobial resistance in the food chain is currently a subject of a major interest. The excessive use or rather misuse of antimicrobials coupled with a poor hygiene in the food production chain has led to a rise of resistant zoonotic bacteria, commonly transmitted by food. They pose a serious threat to human health. Campylobacteriosis is the leading bacterial food-borne illness and most commonly reported zoonosis in humans in the European Union for more than a decade. Salmonellosis is most frequently diagnosed in food-borne outbreaks. Fluoroquinolones are considered as critically important for treatment of severe cases of both zoonoses in humans. Due to an extremely prevalent resistant isolates, especially from broilers and meat, also the treatment of human *Campylobacter* infections with fluoroquinolones has become compromised. *Salmonella* isolates from poultry and poultry meat tend to be highly resistant to fluoroquinolones as well. Beside the resistance to this group of antibiotics, the threat of multiple drug resistant (MDR) *Campylobacter* and *Salmonella* strains is discussed in the light of most recent reports of animal, food and human clinical surveillance systems.

**Keywords:** *Campylobacter*, *Salmonella*, antimicrobial resistance, food safety, food production chain, multiple drug resistance

## 1. Introduction

Antimicrobials are indispensable in human medicine for treating and preventing infectious diseases. In addition, the same classes of antimicrobials are extensively used in livestock not only for the treatment and prevention of infections but also for the growth promotion [1]. The latter has, however, been banned in the European Union (EU) since 2006 [2].

The amounts of antimicrobials utilised in livestock are vast and often exceed those in humans. Data suggest that in the EU approximately 70% of antimicrobials were sold for use in livestock in 2014 [3]. The consumption of antimicrobials in humans and animals has indeed been associated with the occurrence of antimicrobial resistance (AMR) in zoonotic bacteria [3], which are the causative agents of zoonoses and can be transmitted directly between animals and humans or *via* the food chain. AMR in zoonotic bacteria is a subject of major concern.

Even though AMR is an ancient and naturally occurring phenomenon in some bacteria [4], the excessive use of antimicrobials in humans and livestock, as well as poor hygiene conditions and practices in the food production chain, accelerates the emergence of resistance in zoonotic bacteria [5]. The alarming consequence of AMR coupled with the paucity of novel antimicrobials is the rise in the frequency of multidrug resistant (MDR) zoonotic bacteria that may lead to an impaired response to antimicrobial therapy or ultimately even treatment failure [6].

The most current data regarding AMR in zoonotic bacteria are published annually by European Food Safety Authority (EFSA) and European Centre for Disease Control and Prevention (ECDC), but usually with a two-year delay in publishing. According to the recent report on AMR in zoonotic bacteria in 2016 [5], resistance in *Salmonella* and *Campylobacter* is considered of the highest concern. The scope of this review is, therefore, to discuss and emphasise the current trends of AMR in *Salmonella* and *Campylobacter* in the light of the recent EFSA/ECDC report, and the role of whole genome sequencing (WGS) in the surveillance of AMR in *Salmonella* and *Campylobacter* along the food production chain.

## 2. Common zoonoses in Europe

For more than a decade, campylobacteriosis has been the most common zoonosis in Europe. Salmonellosis is the second most commonly reported enteric infection, and the leading cause of food-borne outbreaks. *Campylobacter* and *Salmonella* combined accounted for almost 95% of the reported and confirmed zoonoses cases in 2016 (**Figure 1**).

Salmonellosis is a food-borne gastrointestinal infection caused by zoonotic bacteria *Salmonella* spp. Several thousand serovars of *Salmonella* spp. *enterica* exist, yet only some are causing disease symptoms. Nontyphoidal serovars are transmitted *via* the food chain, whereas typhoidal serovars, the causative agents of typhoid fever, are restricted to humans [8]. Whilst the majority of nontyphoidal *Salmonella* infections are self-limiting and do not require any antibiotic treatment, some cases result in life-threatening systemic infections that must be treated with antimicrobials, primarily fluoroquinolones (FQ) or third-generation cephalosporins [5]. Resistance to these drugs may jeopardise the efficiency of the antimicrobial therapy.

*Campylobacter* spp. are common gut commensals of several animal species, especially birds [9], and the leading cause of gastroenteritis in humans, yet the infections often go unreported. The majority of campylobacterioses are caused by two species, namely *Campylobacter jejuni* and *Campylobacter coli*. Symptoms of campylobacteriosis are also usually mild and self-limiting, although some patients with acute infections that can trigger autoimmune inflammatory conditions need to be treated with antimicrobials, primarily macrolides and FQ [5]. Emergence of resistance in *Campylobacter* is common and thus of concern.

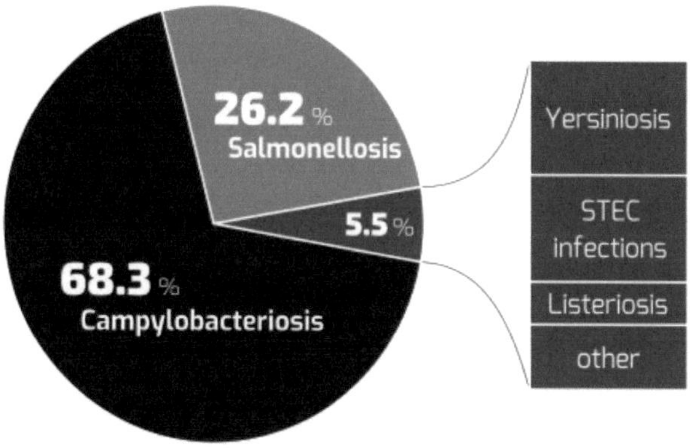


**Figure 1.** Common zoonoses in Europe in 2016. STEC: Shiga toxin-producing *Escherichia coli* [7].

In the Member States (MS) of the EU monitoring and reporting data on zoonoses and AMR for *Salmonella* and *Campylobacter* from animals, food, feed and humans are mandatory [10]. Comparing AMR data from different countries and assessing trends has long been challenging due to inadequate harmonisation of the methodology and reporting among the MS [11]. Recently, great progress has been made in terms of harmonisation of AMR surveillance programs, especially for food animals and foods with the new legislation [12]. In addition, a protocol for harmonised monitoring of AMR in humans has been developed [13], but it is not a legal document that would obligate the MS to its implementation.

## 3. *Salmonella*

### 3.1. Prevalence of nontyphoidal *Salmonella* in the food chain

According to the recent report on trends and sources of zoonoses, zoonotic agents and food-borne outbreaks in 2016 published by EFSA/ECDC [7], the declining trend of salmonellosis in Europe has ended. In 2016, there were 94,530 confirmed cases of salmonellosis with the highest notification rate per 100,000 population in Eastern Europe (in average 46.9 per 100,000), mostly on the account of Czech Republic (110) and Slovakia (97.7), followed by Northern (20.6), Western (18.8) and Southern Europe (13.0). Additionally, *Salmonella* was most regularly detected in food-borne outbreaks (22.3%), which have resulted in the highest burden of hospitalisations (45.6% of the total number of hospitalised cases) and deaths (50% of the total number of deaths among outbreak cases) [7]. Outbreaks were linked to several sources, e.g., Polish eggs [14], infant formula [15] and sesame seeds [16].

*Salmonella* was the most prevalent in meat from turkeys (7.74% of the samples tested positive) and from broilers (6.39%), as well as dried seeds (8.0%) [7], which are an important source of infections, especially due to a long shelf life and low moisture [17]. Chicken, turkey and other avian species are commonly inhabited with *Salmonella* without noticeable symptoms [18], which is in addition to the practices in the food production chain [19], considered the highest risk for contamination of meat products. Even though *Salmonella* was significantly less frequently detected in eggs and their products, they remain the most important source of outbreaks [14, 20], most probably due to a large worldwide consumption coupled with low concentrations of *Salmonella* that cannot be detected [7]. Rapid methods with improved sensitivity are thus needed to address this shortfall, e.g., real-time recombinase polymerase amplification [21] or sequence-based methods.

### 3.2. Antimicrobial resistance in nontyphoidal *Salmonella* spp.

The most recent data (from 2016) on AMR in *Salmonella* from poultry, meat thereof, and humans are provided by EFSA/ECDC [5], whereas data on other livestock are presented in the last-year report [22]. Generally, as shown in **Figure 2**, the isolates of *Salmonella* spp. along the food production chain tend to be highly resistant to tetracyclines and ciprofloxacin (in average in the EU up to 65%), sulfonamides (56%) and ampicillin (45%) with the highest observed frequency in poultry, meat thereof and pigs, respectively (**Figure 2**). Resistance rates seemed to be higher in Southern or Eastern Europe than in Northern or Western Europe [5, 22]. Such extreme rates of resistance that could indeed reflect an extensive use of these three antimicrobials in livestock [23] are of concern and could be facilitating further dissemination of AMR.

Sulfonamides and ampicillin were the former first-line drugs against salmonellosis [24]. Nevertheless, ampicillin, a critically important antimicrobial [25], is used for treating community acquired pneumonia, complicated severe acute malnutrition and sepsis in neonates and children [26]. In contrast, sulfonamides and tetracyclines are classified as highly important antimicrobials [25]. Sulfonamides are the first-line drugs against urinary tract infections and tetracyclines against *Chlamydia trachomatis* and cholera [26].

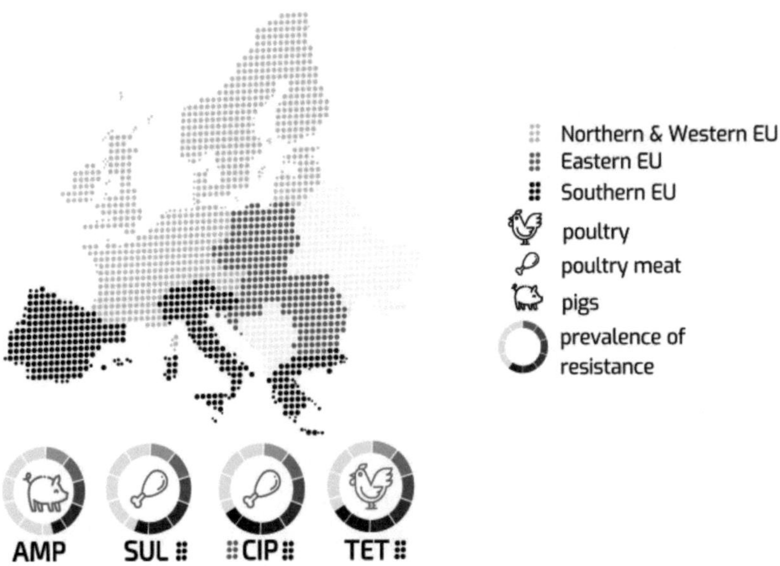


**Figure 2.** Prevalence of resistance in *Salmonella* spp. AMP: ampicillin, SUL: sulfonamides, CIP: ciprofloxacin, TET: tetracyclines [5, 22].

FQ resistance to ciprofloxacin or nalidixic acid that is reflecting similar genetic mechanisms [11] was remarkably high in isolates from poultry meat (**Figure 2**), followed by poultry [5] and has steeply increased since 2004 [27]. That is of concern, because FQ are in addition to third-generation cephalosporins clinically important for the treatment of salmonellosis and several other infections, yet both may be used in livestock.

### 3.3. FQ resistance and third-generation cephalosporins resistance in *Salmonella*

Broiler meat (64.7%), broilers (53.8%), turkey (50.5%) and turkey meat (43.7%) were the main sources of FQ resistance. In contrast, isolates from pigs, humans and laying hens had better susceptibility (**Figure 3**) [5, 22]. The ranges of FQ resistance, however, varied extremely among the countries and even regions. In Spain, for example, isolates from pigs in Catalonia (50%) [28] and humans in Extremadura (35%) [29] exhibited much higher levels of FQ resistance than reported by EFSA/ECDC for Spain (7 and 14.8%, respectively).

FQ resistance in isolates from broilers and meat thereof was in average most prevalent in Southern (62.2, 70.1%, respectively) and Eastern Europe (65.5, 71.5%, respectively) and exceeded 90% in Cyprus, Slovenia and Croatia (**Figure 4**). Of note, only a minority of the MS from Northern Europe reported these data [5]. A rapid increase in FQ resistance is evident in Europe, for instance, in isolates from broilers in Spain resistance increased from 0 [30] to 55.6% in just a few years.

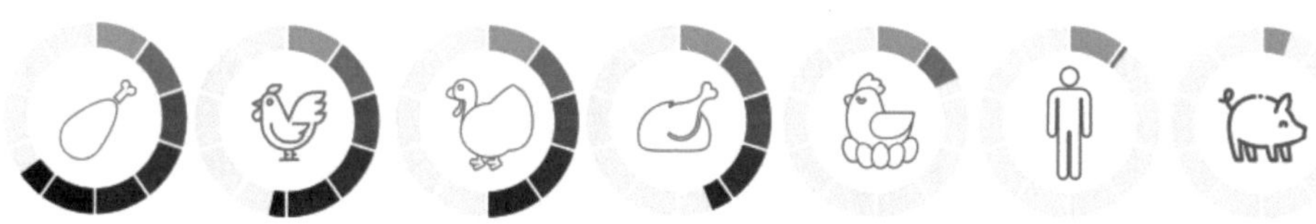

**Figure 3.** Rates of FQ resistance in isolates of *Salmonella* spp. from various sources: broiler meat, broilers, turkeys, turkey meat, laying hens, humans and pigs, respectively [5, 22].

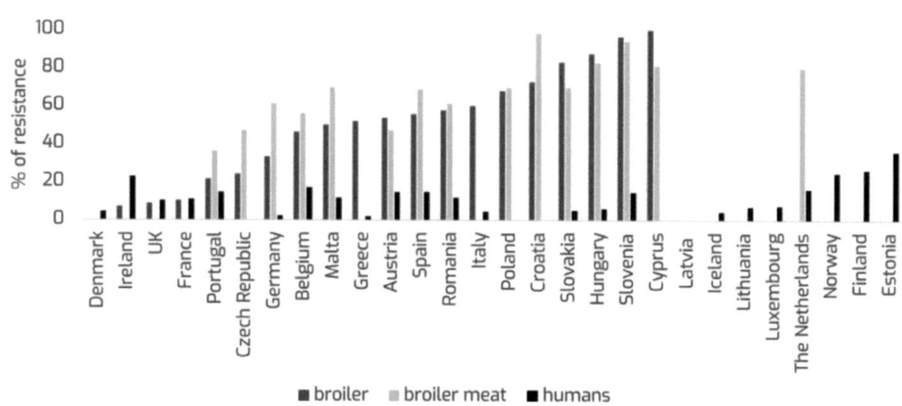


**Figure 4.** Prevalence of FQ-resistant isolates of *Salmonella* spp. from broilers, meat thereof and humans in Europe. UK: United Kingdom [5].

In contrast, the proportions of FQ resistance in humans were significantly lower (11%) [5] and has remained at a relatively stable level since 2009 [31]. The biggest share of FQ resistance was detected in Northern Europe, mostly on the account of Estonia (36.0%), Finland (26.3%), Norway (24.7%) and Ireland (22.9%) (**Figure 4**). Human-associated serovars commonly detected in Europe [32–35] that frequently exhibited FQ resistance were *S.* Infantis (23.4%) and *S.* Kentucky (85.8%) [5].

FQ resistance is a result of a complex mechanism, but it is still not fully understood [36]. Many point mutations in the genes encoding for gyrase and topoisomerase, the two enzymes that are inhibited by FQ, were identified as the causative agents [37]. In addition, plasmids may harbour genes for efflux pumps, target protection proteins or drug-modifying enzymes [38].

Resistance to third-generation cephalosporins was rare in humans as well as in livestock [5], yet when combined with FQ resistance, it poses a serious risk to human health, in terms of reducing the efficiency of these drugs against salmonellosis and thus leaving only the reserve antimicrobials as a feasible therapy option [24]. Resistance to cephalosporins is conferred by genes encoding for AmpC β-lactamase as well as for various extended spectrum β-lactamase (ESBL) that can be located on plasmids. Such isolates were observed in Germany [39] and are assumed to have clonally spread from livestock to humans. Worryingly, in Portugal, more than a third of the isolates from broiler meat (39.4%) exhibited resistance to cefotaxime and ceftazidime and in Italy 12% from broilers [5]. In addition, combined resistance to FQ and cephalosporins was detected in poultry and humans in Spain, Belgium and France [40, 41].

*Salmonella* in the food production chain presents an important reservoir of genetic resistance determinants, which could be mobilised and transferred *via* the food chain to either other human pathogens or commensal bacteria [42]. Notably, importation of meat products [43] and travelling in endemic areas [44], where the rates of resistance to critically important antimicrobials are alarmingly high [45], were linked to the global spread of MDR strains.

### 3.4. MDR and combined resistance to fluoroquinolones and third-generation cephalosporins

In general, 26.5% of the human isolates of *Salmonella* and 50.3% of broiler meat displayed MDR phenotype (defined as resistant to at least three antimicrobials of the nine antimicrobial classes tested). The highest prevalence of MDR isolates from humans was observed in Portugal (51%) and from broiler meat in Slovenia (100%) [5]. MDR strains isolated from pigs in Germany were associated with integrons, which might have an important role in dissemination of resistance [46].

The majority of MDR isolates belonged to serovars *S.* Infantis and *S.* Kentucky. Among human isolates of *S.* Kentucky, which is the seventh most common serovar, MDR was recorded at extremely high levels (76.3%) [5]. *S.* Kentucky ST198 clone that is displaying high-level resistance to ciprofloxacin and frequently also to amoxicillin, streptomycin, spectinomycin, gentamicin, sulfamethoxazole and tetracycline has been imported from North Africa and has been widely spread across Europe in humans and food production chain [32]. In addition, acquisition of extended-spectrum β-lactamase, plasmid-encoded cephalosporinase or carbapenemase in this clone was detected in Mediterranean area [47] and in Poland [33]. Combined resistance was also detected in *S.* Kentucky from humans and livestock in Belgium, Luxembourg, Malta, the Netherlands and Germany [5].

*S.* Infantis was the most prevalent serovar in broilers and the fourth among human infections. Multi-drug resistance to FQ, sulfonamides and tetracyclines was observed frequently in the isolates from broilers (75.3%), broiler meat (72.6%), as well as in isolates from humans in two MS (Austria and Slovenia) that together with Hungary and Croatia accounted for a majority of the *S.* Infantis isolates from broilers. This indicates the presence of a specific MDR clone prevalent in this geographical region [5]. In addition, resistance to cephalosporins was recorded in the isolates from either humans, food or poultry in Great Britain [48], Switzerland [34], Italy [35], as well as in the USA [49], in some cases located on a plasmid and thus conferring a risk of transfer. Such strains can be transmitted from broilers and broiler meat to humans and may lead to human infections [35].

## 4. *Campylobacter*

### 4.1. Prevalence of *Campylobacter* in the food chain

Whilst *Campylobacter,* with 246,307 confirmed infections in 2016 and 6.1% increase relative to 2015, accounted for the majority of zoonoses in Europe, the death toll was low (0.03%). The highest notification rate per 100,000 population was observed in Eastern Europe (71.4), followed by Western (65.7), Southern (56.3) and Northern Europe (55.0). Czech Republic (228.2) and Slovakia (140.5) were the countries with the highest prevalence [7].

Campylobacters were most frequently detected in turkeys (65.3%) and meat thereof (11%) as well as in broilers (27.3%) and meat thereof (36.7%) [7], making the poultry food production chain the main source of contamination. This is in concordance to data from several reports [50, 51]. The prevalence in retail poultry meat was, however, reported even up to almost 90% [50]. *Campylobacter* was also detected in cattle [52], pigs [53] and sheep [54]. Contaminated farm environment or equipment as well as the presence of *Campylobacter* in other animals and wildlife, were significantly associated with the prevalence of *Campylobacter* in poultry [55]. Furthermore, recent data suggest that human clinical *C. jejuni* isolates in Central Europe can be attributed to domesticated poultry, cattle livestock and environmental sources [56].

Outbreaks can be traced back to several sources (e.g., raw milk [57], water [58] and chicken liver pate [59]) and even associated with antimicrobial-resistant strains [57]. However, a limited number of highly contaminated products are most probably responsible for the majority of *Campylobacter* infections. Effective and harmonised surveillance systems, especially in the poultry food production chain, that are oriented towards categorising risks should thus be established [50].

### 4.2. Antimicrobial resistance in *Campylobacter*

*Campylobacter* spp. in 2016 displayed extremely high resistance levels to FQ, which is particularly worrisome, as FQ are used as the first-line drugs against campylobacteriosis. Consequently, in some EU countries, FQ therapy of campylobacteriosis is no longer feasible. In average, the highest share of resistant isolates was detected in poultry and meat thereof, especially in the Member States of Southern and Eastern Europe (**Figure 5**) [5]. Data suggest that the use of FQ in livestock, specifically pigs, selects for FQ-resistant strains and accelerates the dissemination of such strains [60].

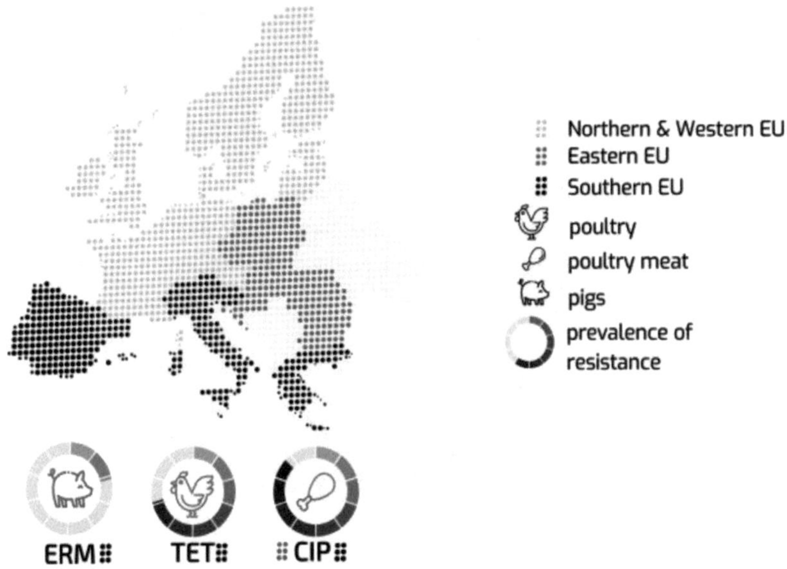


**Figure 5.** Prevalence of resistance in *Campylobacter* spp. ERM: erythromycin, CIP: ciprofloxacin, TET: tetracyclines [5, 22].

In general, resistance to erythromycin, the second clinically important antimicrobial for treating campylobacteriosis, is generally uncommon; however, more resistant isolates were detected in pigs (21.6% in 2015), as seen in **Figure 5** [22], which could reflect a wide use of macrolides for the treatment of common infections in pigs [61]. In contrast to *C. jejuni* from humans (2.1%), markedly higher erythromycin resistance level was observed in *C. coli* (11.0%), with the highest proportion in Estonia (63.2%) and Portugal (50%). Similar trends could be observed in isolates from livestock and food [5]. Similarly, high levels of resistance (62.4%) were recorded in *C. coli* from pigs in Spain [22] and even higher in *Campylobacter* isolates from poultry meat in Italy (72.1%) [62].

Resistance to macrolides in *Campylobacter* most commonly occurs *via* chromosomal mutations in 23S rRNA [63] that reduces the binding affinity of macrolides to the binding site. These mutations were, however, demonstrated to have a fitness cost and to slow growth rates [64]. Recently, transferrable erythromycin resistance, conferred by the rRNA methylase *erm(B)* gene and located on either plasmids or associated with chromosomal multidrug resistance genomic islands, was detected in humans and livestock [65].

Southern Europe in average recorded higher prevalence of resistance to tetracyclines, which may also be used for the treatment of campylobacteriosis in humans, and is, in addition to FQ resistance, a very common feature [5]. Marked variations in tetracycline resistance could be observed between *C. coli* and *C. jejuni,* countries and sources of isolation. Resistance rates varied from very low (<10%) in *C. coli* from pigs in Sweden [66], moderate in *Campylobacter* spp. from cattle in Poland (20.9%) [52], *C. jejuni* from broiler carcasses in Belgium (47%) [67] and *C. jejuni* from chicken meat in France (53.6%) [51] to extremely high in isolates of *C. coli* from pigs in France (93%) [66], as well as *Campylobacter* spp. from quails in Portugal (96.7%) [68]. In general, *C. coli* exhibited higher resistance levels [5].

### 4.3. FQ resistance and combined/MDR resistance in *Campylobacter*

FQ resistance first emerged in Southeast Asia early in the 1990s with a rapid increase from 0 to 84% over the period of 4 years [69] and has been widely spread to the other parts of the world, which might be due to an enhanced fitness of FQ-resistant isolates [70]. Significant portion of infections with FQ-resistant *Campylobacter* could be acquired through travel [71]. Extreme rates of FQ resistance in endemic areas [72] are therefore of concern.

In Europe, FQ resistance in *Campylobacter* spp. was extremely high, but it varied among the sources of isolation, species and countries. In average, isolates of *C. coli* exhibited markedly higher resistance rates than isolates of *C. jejuni*. As seen in **Figure 6**, turkey (96.8% in *C. coli* and 76.2% in *C. jejuni*) and meat thereof (100% in *C. coli*, 74.5% in *C. jejuni*) presented the main sources of resistance, closely followed by broilers and meat thereof [5].

A rapid increase in FQ resistance in *Campylobacter* is evident in the last 14 years [27]. In Slovenia, for instance, the resistance level to nalidixic acid rapidly increased in isolates from broiler meat from 49.1% in 2001–2003 [73] to 78.6% in 2006 [11]. In 2016, in average, 77.3% of *Campylobacter* spp. from broilers exhibited FQ resistance [5]. Recent data suggest the presence and clonal spread of FQ-resistant *C. jejuni* clonal complex ST-21 in central Europe (Slovenia, Germany, Austria) [74].

FQ resistance in *C. jejuni* (**Figure 7**) from broilers (in average 66.9%) varied from 8.4% in Finland to 97.9% in Latvia [5]. Furthermore, in 2014, Latvia reported on 100% resistant isolates

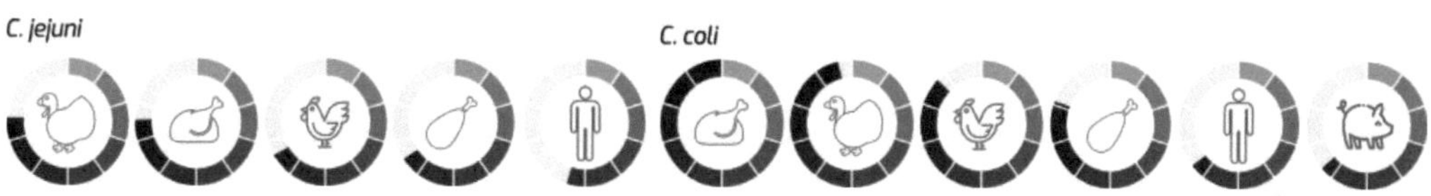


**Figure 6.** Sources and prevalence of FQ-resistant isolates of *C. jejuni* (turkey, turkey meat, broilers, broiler meat and human, respectively) and *C. coli* (turkey meat, turkeys, broilers, broiler meat, humans and pigs, respectively) [5, 22].

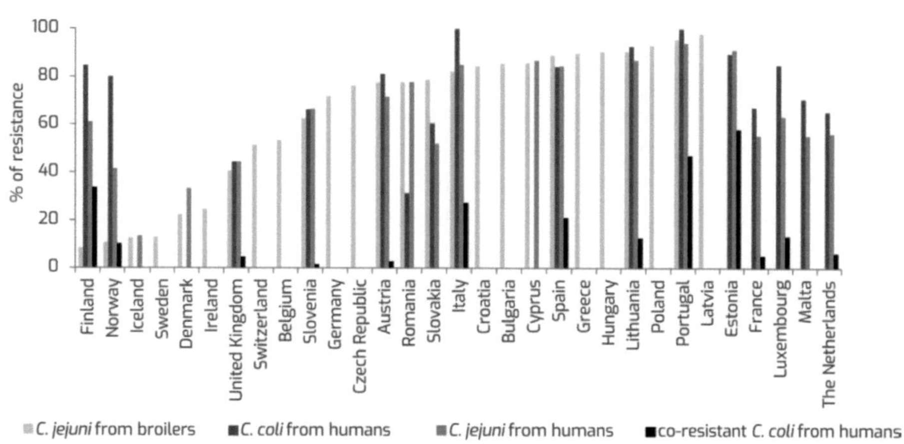


**Figure 7.** Rates of FQ resistance in *C. jejuni* from broilers and humans, in *C. coli* from humans and combined resistance to FQ and erythromycin in *C. coli* from humans [5].

of *Campylobacter* from chicken [75]. In humans, the highest rates of FQ resistance were reported for *C. coli* from Italy and Portugal (100%) and in for *C. jejuni* from Portugal and Estonia (>90%). Notably, 9 out of 19 EU MS recorded 80–100% resistance rates for *C. coli* (**Figure 7**) [5].

Overall, 9.2% of human *C. coli* exhibited combined resistance to ciprofloxacin, erythromycin and tetracycline with resistance rates ranging from 0 to 57.9% (Estonia), which is shown in **Figure 7** [5]. Erythromycin resistance is often associated with MDR phenotype [63]. In Finland, for example, 94.7% of *Campylobacter* isolates from humans were, in addition to erythromycin, resistant to FQ, and 73.7% to tetracycline [76]. Combined resistance to the first-line drugs may be associated with adverse events such as delayed recovery, invasive illness and prolonged treatment with feasible alternative antimicrobials [77, 78].

FQ resistance in *C. jejuni* and *C. coli* can be mediated through specific point mutations in *gyrA* gene, encoding for DNA gyrase or through chromosomally encoded multidrug efflux pump. The two mechanisms work synergistically [79]. Efflux pumps in *Campylobacter*, primarily CmeABC, are involved in resistance to broad spectrum of antimicrobials, including macrolides and quinolones [80], as well as cross-resistance to other compounds such as bile salts [81]. Therapeutic application of efflux pump inhibitors (e.g., epigallocatechin gallate) that were shown to restore macrolide efficacy could be a feasible treatment option in combination with the macrolide therapy [80, 82–84].

## 5. The role of whole genome sequencing in the surveillance of antimicrobial resistance of common zoonotic bacteria

The EU harmonised system on the monitoring and reporting of antimicrobial resistance in zoonotic and commensal bacteria (EC Decision 2013/652/EU; EFSA, EDSA) [12] is based on the phenotypic assessment of AMR of selected bacterial species (*Salmonella, Campylobacter, E. coli*) in selected food-producing animal species (poultry, pigs, cattle) and food products (chicken, pork, beef meat), using dilution methods (ISO standard 20776-1:2006, ISO standard 20776-2:2007) and EUCAST epidemiological cut-off values (ECOFF-values) as interpretative criteria (EC Decision 2013/652/EU) [12]. In accordance with this legislation, 170 isolates are examined for antimicrobial susceptibility to a panel of 15 antimicrobial substances, for each combination of bacterial species and type of sample of animal population or food category each year by each member state. In 2016, ECDC also published EU protocol for harmonised monitoring of antimicrobial resistance in human *Salmonella* and *Campylobacter* isolates, aimed to increase the comparability of AMR data collected at the EU level from different Member States, and to improve the comparison of data among human isolates and isolates from animals and food products [13]. Beside dilution method as a preferred method, disk diffusion and gradient strip diffusion method are also allowed.

On the isolate level, genotyping of human isolates is also recommended, in terms of the assessment of resistance mechanisms and detection of the epidemic spread of resistance, particularly multi-drug resistant *Salmonella*, but it is not required in reporting [13].

In recent years, the development of high-throughput technologies and platforms for massive DNA sequencing, and genomics tools has opened new possibilities also in the surveillance of AMR in common zoonotic bacteria. WGS, together with appropriate databases, general (NCBI, ENA) or specialised for AMR (ARG-ANNOT, ResFinder, CARD, RED-DB, Bacmet), bioinformatic tools (BLAST) and platforms enable detection of antibiotic resistance genetic loci in the genomes of bacterial isolates or microbiomes and reveal the mechanisms leading to AMR. While WGS offers very rapid and efficient tool for detection of the antibiotic resistance genes (ARG) in genomes of individual bacterial isolates, the main issue remains how to predict from these data the actual antimicrobial susceptibility, and epidemiological or clinical cut-off values [85]. However, differentiation among isolates with acquired or intrinsic resistance on the basis of phenotypic MIC determinations only is also not totally accurate. Furthermore, it should be considered that also the strains that contain the genes associated with antimicrobial resistance but do not exhibit phenotypic resistance present certain risk for the horizontal spread when consumed.

The usefulness of WGS for antimicrobial resistance surveillance was confirmed in several studies. Examination of 640 nontyphoidal *Salmonella* isolates from retail meat and human clinical samples identified known resistance genes and phenotypic resistance to 14 antimicrobials, where the correlation between resistance genotypes and phenotypes was close to 100% for most classes of antibiotics, and lower for aminoglycosides and beta-lactams [86]. In addition to known ARG, several unique resistance genes were found, more in the human isolates (n = 59) than in the retail meat isolates (n = 36). The authors concluded that the use of more appropriate MIC breakpoints and inclusion of new AGSs in the databases will further improve the correlations between phenotypic and genotypic observations. For *Salmonella typhimurium* isolates (n = 50) from Danish pigs, high concordance (99.74%) between phenotypic and predicted antimicrobial susceptibility was observed as well [87]. Phenotypic resistance to quinolones and fluoroquinolones due to chromosomal mutations, however, could not be detected by ResFinder platform.

Genomic approach is increasingly used also in the developing of control methods and identification of antimicrobial resistance markers for evidence-based decisions in epidemiology and surveillance of foodborne diseases. OMICS datasets have been found as a powerful tool to complement current studies that are starting to be used also in some risk assessment areas. In a current comprehensive study "Syst-OMICS," 4500 *Salmonella* genomes will be sequenced and analysis pipeline built in order to study *Salmonella* genome evolution, antibiotic resistance and virulence genes [88]. The data of the first 3377 genomes already sequenced are stored in the newly established *Salmonella* Foodborne Syst-OMICS database (SalFoS, https://salfos.ibis.ulaval.ca/). Their analysis identified 1003 unique resistomes, composed of combinations of 195 different genes. Surprisingly, the two most frequently observed resistomes accounted for 23% of the *Salmonella* strains examined.

Comparative genomics of the WGS was successfully used also in the examination of 589 *Campylobacter* isolates from retail chicken meat exhibiting phenotypic resistance to 9 antimicrobials [89]. For most antimicrobial agents (ciprofloxacin, nalidixic acid, gentamicin, azithromycin, erythromycin and clindamycin), the observed phenotypic resistance, determined on the basis of the comparison of measured MICs with established ECOFF cut-off values, was in accordance with the presence of the known resistance genes or mutations. In the case of telithromycin, however, the observed point mutations in the 23S rRNA, which is a well-known mechanism of resistance to these classes of antimicrobials, did not regularly cause phenotypic resistance. Another recent study on C. *jejuni* isolates from the poultry (n = 502) demonstrated successful use of genomics in the study of fluoroquinolone resistance [90]. The isolates were clustered according to the presence/absence of the *gyrA* mutations causing fluoroquinolone resistance. Beside the WGS of isolates from the mentioned study, previously published (ENA) *Campylobacter* genomes were included in the comparative analyses of the genomes. Although no significant associations were found between trade patterns, antimicrobial use in livestock and population of *C. jejuni*, this approach proved to be successful, especially when big datasets are available.

In conclusion, comparative genomics of WGS is increasingly used in the prediction of phenotypic antimicrobial resistance and surveillance of antimicrobial resistance of common zoonotic bacteria. However, as it is based on the detection of already known ARG, the success is highly dependent on the quality of databases, which need to be regularly updated with newly discovered resistance mechanisms and well-curated.

## 6. Conclusion

Antimicrobial resistant zoonotic bacteria pose a serious risk to human health. High rates of FQ resistance in both *Salmonella* and *Campylobacter* are of concern due to their wide use for the treatment of human infections. In some regions of the EU, the level of FQ resistance is so high that *Campylobacter* infections cannot be treated with FQ anymore. In addition, the emergence of multi-drug resistant *Salmonella* and *Campylobacter* further limits the therapy options and is possibly associated with adverse treatment effects. Greater efforts are needed to limit the wide spread of AMR in zoonotic bacteria—implementation of antimicrobial stewardship, especially in the developing countries, development of novel antimicrobials, improvement of practices in the food production chain, reduction of the amounts of antimicrobials sold for use in livestock, improvement of AMR surveillance programs, in terms of greater harmonisation, and application of rapid sequence-based methods in the routine surveillance of antimicrobial resistance.

## Acknowledgements

This work was supported by the Slovenian Research Agency (ARRS) through the Research program P4-0116 (Microbiology and Biotechnology of Food and Environment) and P4-0097 (Nutrition and Microbial Ecology of Gastrointestinal Tract).

## Conflict of interest

No competing financial interests exist.

## Author details

Vita Rozman, Bojana Bogovič Matijašić and Sonja Smole Možina*

*Address all correspondence to: sonja.smole@bf.uni-lj.si

Biotechnical Faculty, University of Ljubljana, Slovenia

## References

[1] World Health Organisation. Tackling Antibiotic Resistance from a Food Safety Perspective in Europe. [Internet]. Copenhagen: World Health Organization; 2011. p. 65. Available from: http://www.euro.who.int/__data/assets/pdf_file/0005/136454/e94889.pdf?ua=1

[2] European Commision. Ban on Antibiotics as Growth Promoters in Animal Feed Enters into Effect. [Internet]. 2006. Available from: http://europa.eu/rapid/press-release_IP-05-1687_en.htm [Accessed: 14-06-2018]

[3] ECDC/EFSA/EMA. ECDC/EFSA/EMA second joint report on the integrated analysis of the consumption of antimicrobial agents and occurrence of antimicrobial resistance in bacteria from humans and food-producing animals. EFSA Journal. 2017;**15**:4872. DOI: 10.2903/j.efsa.2017.4872

[4] D'Costa VM, King CE, Kalan L, Morar M, Sung WWL, Schwarz C, et al. Antibiotic resistance is ancient. Nature. 2011;**477**:457-461. DOI: 10.1038/nature10388

[5] EFSA/ECDC. The European Union summary report on antimicrobial resistance in zoonotic and indicator bacteria from humans, animals and food in 2016. EFSA Journal. 2018;**16**:5182. DOI: 10.2903/j.efsa.2018.5182

[6] WHO. Antimicrobial resistance. Global report on surveillance. Bulletin of the World Health Organization. 2014;**61**:383-394. DOI: 10.1007/s13312-014-0374-3

[7] EFSA/ECDC. The European Union summary report on trends and sources of zoonoses, zoonotic agents and food-borne outbreaks in 2016. EFSA Journal. 2017;**15**:5077. DOI: 10.2903/j.efsa.2017.5077

[8] Haraga A, Ohlson MB, Miller SI. Salmonellae interplay with host cells. Nature Reviews. Microbiology. 2008;**6**:53-66. DOI: 10.1038/nrmicro1788

[9] Bolton DJ. *Campylobacter* virulence and survival factors. Food Microbiology. 2015;**48**: 99-108. DOI: 10.1016/j.fm.2014.11.017

[10] European Parliament and Council. Directive 2003/99/EC of the European Parliament and of the Council of 17 November 2003 on the monitoring of zoonoses and zoonotic agents, amending Council Decision 90/424/EEC and repealing Council Directive 92/117/EEC. Official Journal of the European Union [Internet]. 2003;**325**:31-40. Available from: https://eur-lex.europa.eu/legal-content/EN/TXT/?uri=celex%3A32003L0099

[11] Smole Možina S, Kurinčič M, Klančnik A, Mavri A. *Campylobacter* and its multi-resistance in the food chain. Trends in Food Science and Technology. 2011;**22**:91-98. DOI: 10.1016/j.tifs.2010.09.003

[12] European Parliament and Council. Commission Implementing Decision 2013/652/EU of 12 November 2013 on the monitoring and reporting of antimicrobial resistance in zoonotic and commensal bacteria. Official Journal of the European Union [Internet]. 2013;**56**:26-39. Available from: https://publications.europa.eu/en/publication-detail/-/publication/83e1934f-4d39-11e3-ae03-01aa75ed71a1/language-en

[13] ECDC. EU Protocol for Harmonised Monitoring of Antimicrobial Resistance in Human *Salmonella* and *Campylobacter* Isolates. ECDC: Stockholm; 2016. DOI: 10.2900/516074

[14] ECDC/EFSA. Multi-Country Outbreak of *Salmonella* Enteritidis Infections Linked to Polish Eggs. Stockholm and Parma: ECDC and EFSA; 2017. DOI: 10.2903/sp.efsa.2017.EN-1353

[15] ECDC/EFSA. Multi-Country Outbreak of *Salmonella* Agona Linked to Infant Formula. Stockholm and Parma: ECDC and EFSA; 2018. DOI: 10.2903/sp.efsa.2018.EN-1365

[16] ECDC/EFSA. Multi-Country Outbreak of New *Salmonella enterica* 11:z41:e ,n,z15 Infections Associated with Sesame Seeds. Stockholm and Parma: ECDC/EFSA; 2017. DOI: 10.2903/sp.efsa.2017.EN-1256

[17] Garces-Vega F, Jeong S, Dolan K, Marks B. Modeling *Salmonella* inactivation in low moisture foods: Using parameter estimation to improve model performance. Procedia Food Science. 2016;**7**:41-46. DOI: 10.1016/j.profoo.2016.02.083

[18] Antunes P, Mourão J, Campos J, Peixe L. Salmonellosis: The role of poultry meat. Clinical Microbiology and Infection. 2015;**22**:110-121. DOI: 10.1016/j.cmi.2015.12.004

[19] Rouger A, Tresse O, Zagorec M. Bacterial contaminants of poultry meat: Sources, species, and dynamics. Microorganisms. 2017;**5**:16. DOI: 10.3390/microorganisms5030050

[20] Chousalkar K, Gast R, Martelli F, Pande V. Review of egg-related salmonellosis and reduction strategies in United States, Australia, United Kingdom and New Zealand. Critical Reviews in Microbiology. 2018;**44**:290-303. DOI: 10.1080/1040841X.2017.1368998

[21] Kim JY, Lee JL. Rapid detection of *Salmonella enterica* serovar Enteritidis from eggs and chicken meat by real-time recombinase polymerase amplification in comparison with the two-step real-time PCR. Journal of Food Safety. 2016;**36**:402-411. DOI: 10.1111/jfs.12261

[22] EFSA/ECDC. The European Union summary report on antimicrobial resistance in zoonotic and indicator bacteria from humans, animals and food in 2015. EFSA Journal. 2017;**15**:4694. DOI: 10.2903/j.efsa.2017.4694

[23] EMA. Sales of Veterinary Antimicrobial Agents in 29 European Countries in 2014 [Internet]. 2016. p. 176. Available from: http://www.ema.europa.eu/docs/en_GB/document_library/Report/2016/10/WC500214217.pdf; DOI: 10.2809/676974

[24] Kleine CE, Schlabe S, Hischebeth GTR, Molitor E, Pfeifer Y, Wasmuth JC, et al. Successful therapy of a multidrug-resistant extended-spectrum β-lactamase-producing and fluoroquinolone-resistant *Salmonella enterica* subspecies enterica Serovar Typhi infection using combination therapy of meropenem and fosfomycin. Clinical Infectious Diseases. 2017;**65**:1754-1756. DOI: 10.1093/cid/cix652

[25] WHO. Critically Important Antimicrobials for Human Medicine. 5th rev ed. Geneva: World Health Organization (WHO); 2017. 42 p. DOI: 10.1017/CBO9781107415324.004

[26] WHO. WHO Model List of Essential Medicines. 20th ed. Geneva: WHO; 2017. 39 p. DOI: 10.1016/S1473-3099(14)70780-7

[27] EFSA/ECDC. The European Union summary report on antimicrobial resistance in zoonotic and indicator bacteria from humans, animals and food in 2004-2007. EFSA Journal. 2009;**8**:1309. DOI: 10.2903/j.efsa.2010.1309

[28] Cameron-Veas K, Fraile L, Napp S, Garrido V, Grilló MJ, Migura-Garcia L. Multidrug resistant *Salmonella enterica* isolated from conventional pig farms using antimicrobial agents in preventative medicine programmes. Veterinary Journal. 2018;**234**:36-42. DOI: 10.1016/j.tvjl.2018.02.002

[29] Campos MJ, Palomo G, Hormeño L, Herrera-León S, Domínguez L, Vadillo S, et al. Prevalence of quinolone resistance determinants in non-typhoidal *Salmonella* isolates from human origin in Extremadura, Spain. Diagnostic Microbiology and Infectious Disease. 2014;**79**:64-69. DOI: 10.1016/j.diagmicrobio.2014.01.010

[30] Lamas A, Fernandez-No IC, Miranda JM, Vázquez B, Cepeda A, Franco CM. Prevalence, molecular characterization and antimicrobial resistance of *Salmonella* serovars isolated from northwestern Spanish broiler flocks (2011-2015). Poultry Science. 2016;**95**:2097-2105. DOI: 10.3382/ps/pew150

[31] EFSA/ECDC. The European Union Summary Report on antimicrobial resistance in antimicrobial resistance in zoonotic and indicator bacteria from humans, animals and food in the European Union in 2009. EFSA Journal. 2011;**9**:2154. DOI: 10.2903/j.efsa.2011.2154

[32] Le Hello S, Hendriksen RS, Doublet B, Fisher I, Nielsen EM, Whichard JM, et al. International spread of an epidemic population of *Salmonella enterica* serotype Kentucky ST198 resistant to ciprofloxacin. The Journal of Infectious Diseases. 2011;**204**:675-684. DOI: 10.1093/infdis/jir409

[33] Wasyl D, Kern-Zdanowicz I, Domańska-Blicharz K, Zajac M, Hoszowski A. High-level fluoroquinolone resistant *Salmonella enterica* serovar Kentucky ST198 epidemic clone with IncA/C conjugative plasmid carrying blaCTX-M-25 gene. Veterinary Microbiology. 2015;**175**:85-91. DOI: 10.1016/j.vetmic.2014.10.014

[34] Hindermann D, Gopinath G, Chase H, Negrete F, Althaus D, Zurfluh K, et al. *Salmonella enterica* serovar Infantis from food and human infections, Switzerland, 2010-2015: Poultry-related multidrug resistant clones and an emerging ESBL producing clonal lineage. Frontiers in Microbiology. 2017;**8**:1322. DOI: 10.3389/fmicb.2017.01322

[35] Franco A, Leekitcharoenphon P, Feltrin F, Alba P, Cordaro G, Iurescia M, et al. Emergence of a clonal lineage of multidrug-resistant ESBL-producing *Salmonella* infantis transmitted from broilers and broiler meat to humans in Italy between 2011 and 2014. PLoS One. 2015;**10**:e0144802. DOI: 10.1371/journal.pone.0144802

[36] Correia S, Hébraud M, Poeta P, Capelo JL, Igrejas G. How combined multicomparative proteomic approaches can improve the understanding of quinolone resistance in *Salmonella* Typhimurium. Future Microbiology. 2018;**13**:403-406. DOI: 10.2217/fmb-2017-0250

[37] Mąka Ł, Maćkiw E, Stasiak M, Wołkowicz T, Kowalska J, Postupolski J, et al. Ciprofloxacin and nalidixic acid resistance of *Salmonella* spp. isolated from retail food in Poland. International Journal of Food Microbiology. 2018;**276**:1-4. DOI: 10.1016/j.ijfoodmicro.2018.03.012

[38] Correia S, Poeta P, Hébraud M, Capelo JL, Igrejas G. Mechanisms of quinolone action and resistance: Where do we stand? Journal of Medical Microbiology. 2017;**66**:551-559. DOI: 10.1099/jmm.0.000475

[39] Eller C, Simon S, Miller T, Frick JS, Prager R, Rabsch W, et al. Presence of β-lactamases in extended-spectrum-cephalosporinresistant *Salmonella enterica* of 30 different serovars in Germany 2005-11. The Journal of Antimicrobial Chemotherapy. 2013;**68**:1978-1981. DOI: 10.1093/jac/dkt163

[40] Machuca J, Agüero J, Miró E, Del Carmen CM, Oteo J, Bou G, et al. Prevalence of quinolone resistance mechanisms in Enterobacteriaceae producing acquired AmpC β-lactamases and/or carbapenemases in Spain. Enfermedades Infecciosas y Microbiología Clínica. 2017;**35**:485-490. DOI: 10.1016/j.eimc.2016.05.006

[41] Bertrand S, Weill FX, Cloeckaert A, Vrints M, Mairiaux E, Fraud K, et al. Clonal emergence of extended-spectrum β-lactamase (CTX-M-2)-producing *Salmonella enterica* serovar virchow isolates with reduced susceptibilities to ciprofloxacin among poultry and humans in Belgium and France (2000-2003). Journal of Clinical Microbiology. 2006;**44**:2897-2903. DOI: 10.1128/JCM.02549-05

[42] Card RM, Cawthraw SA, Nunez-Garcia J, Ellis RJ, Kay G, Pallen MJ, et al. An in vitro chicken gut model demonstrates transfer of a multidrug resistance plasmid from *Salmonella* to commensal *Escherichia coli*. mBio. 2017;**8**:e00777-e00717. DOI: 10.1128/mBio.00777-17

[43] Campos J, Mourão J, Silveira L, Saraiva M, Correia CB, Maçãs AP, et al. Imported poultry meat as a source of extended-spectrum cephalosporin-resistant CMY-2-producing *Salmonella* Heidelberg and *Salmonella* Minnesota in the European Union, 2014-2015. International Journal of Antimicrobial Agents. 2018;**51**:151-154. DOI: 10.1016/j.ijantimicag.2017.09.006

[44] Ferstl PG, Reinheimer C, Jozsa K, Zeuzem S, Kempf VAJ, Waidmann O, et al. Severe infection with multidrug-resistant *Salmonella* choleraesuis in a young patient with primary sclerosing cholangitis. World Journal of Gastroenterology. 2017;**23**:2086-2089. DOI: 10.3748/wjg.v23.i11.2086

[45] Jiang HX, Song L, Liu J, Zhang XH, Ren YN, Zhang WH, et al. Multiple transmissible genes encoding fluoroquinolone and third-generation cephalosporin resistance co-located in non-typhoidal *Salmonella* isolated from food-producing animals in China. International Journal of Antimicrobial Agents. 2014;**43**:242-247. DOI: 10.1016/j.ijantimicag.2013.12.005

[46] Argüello H, Guerra B, Rodr I, Rubio P, Carvajal A. Characterization of antimicrobial resistance determinants and class 1 and class 2 integrons in *Salmonella* enterica spp., multidrug-resistant isolates from pigs. Genes (Basel). 2018;**16**:E256. DOI: 10.3390/genes9050256

[47] Le Hello S, Harrois D, Bouchrif B, Sontag L, Elhani D, Guibert V, et al. Highly drug-resistant *Salmonella* enterica serotype Kentucky ST198-X1: A microbiological study. The Lancet Infectious Diseases. 2013;**13**:672-679. DOI: 10.1016/S1473-3099(13)70124-5

[48] Burke L, Hopkins KL, Meunier D, De Pinna E, Fitzgerald-Hughes D, Humphreys H, et al. Resistance to third-generation cephalosporins in human non-typhoidal *Salmonella* enterica isolates from England and Wales, 2010-12. The Journal of Antimicrobial Chemotherapy. 2014;**69**:977-981. DOI: 10.1093/jac/dkt469

[49] Tate H, Folster JP, Hsu CH, Chen J, Hoffmann M, Li C, et al. Comparative analysis of extended-spectrum-β-lactamase CTX-M-65-producing *Salmonella* enterica serovar infantis isolates from humans, food animals, and retail chickens in the United States. Antimicrobial Agents and Chemotherapy. 2017;**61**:e00488-e00417. DOI: 10.1128/AAC.00488-17

[50] Stella S, Soncini G, Ziino G, Panebianco A, Pedonese F, Nuvoloni R, et al. Prevalence and quantification of thermophilic *Campylobacter* spp. in Italian retail poultry meat: Analysis of influencing factors. Food Microbiology. 2017;**62**:232-238. DOI: 10.1016/j.fm.2016.10.028

[51] Guyard-Nicodème M, Rivoal K, Houard E, Rose V, Quesne S, Mourand G, et al. Prevalence and characterization of *Campylobacter jejuni* from chicken meat sold in French retail outlets. International Journal of Food Microbiology. 2015;**203**:8-14. DOI: 10.1016/j.ijfoodmicro.2015.02.013

[52] Wieczorek K, Denis E, Lynch O, Osek J. Molecular characterization and antibiotic resistance profiling of *Campylobacter* isolated from cattle in Polish slaughterhouses. Food Microbiology. 2013;**34**:130-136. DOI: 10.1016/j.fm.2012.12.003

[53] Morales-Partera AM, Cardoso-Toset F, Luque I, Astorga RJ, Maldonado A, Herrera-León S, et al. Prevalence and diversity of *Salmonella* spp., *Campylobacter* spp., and *Listeria monocytogenes* in two free-range pig slaughterhouses. Food Control. 2018;**92**:208-215. DOI: 10.1016/j.foodcont.2018.04.053

[54] Yang R, Jacobson C, Gardner G, Carmichael I, Campbell AJD, Ryan U. Longitudinal prevalence, faecal shedding and molecular characterisation of *Campylobacter* spp. and *Salmonella* enterica in sheep. Veterinary Journal. 2014;**202**:250-254. DOI: 10.1016/j.tvjl.2014.08.001

[55] Ellis-Iversen J, Ridley A, Morris V, Sowa A, Harris J, Atterbury R, et al. Persistent environmental reservoirs on farms as risk factors for *Campylobacter* in commercial poultry. Epidemiology and Infection. 2012;**140**:916-924. DOI: 10.1017/S095026881100118X

[56] Kovač J, Stessl B, Čadež N, Gruntar I, Cimerman M, Stingl K, et al. Population structure and attribution of human clinical *Campylobacter jejuni* isolates from central Europe to livestock and environmental sources. Zoonoses and Public Health. 2018;**65**:51-58. DOI: 10.1111/zph.12366

[57] Burakoff A, Brown K, Knutsen J, Hopewell C, Rowe S, Bennett C, et al. Outbreak of fluoroquinolone-resistant *Campylobacter jejuni* infections associated with raw milk consumption from a herdshare dairy—Colorado, 2016. Morbidity and Mortality Weekly Report. 2018;**67**:146-148. DOI: 10.15585/mmwr.mm6705a2

[58] Revez J, Llarena AK, Schott T, Kuusi M, Hakkinen M, Kivistö R, et al. Genome analysis of *Campylobacter jejuni* strains isolated from a waterborne outbreak. BMC Genomics. 2014;**15**:768. DOI: 10.1186/1471-2164-15-768

[59] Lahti E, Löfdahl M, Agren J, Hansson I, Olsson EE. Confirmation of a campylobacteriosis outbreak associated with chicken liver pate using PFGE and WGS. Zoonoses and Public Health. 2017;**64**:14-20. DOI: 10.1111/zph.12272

[60] Usui M, Sakemi Y, Uchida I, Tamura Y. Effects of fluoroquinolone treatment and group housing of pigs on the selection and spread of fluoroquinolone-resistant *Campylobacter*. Veterinary Microbiology. 2014;**170**:438-441. DOI: 10.1016/j.vetmic.2014.01.036

[61] Pyörälä S, Baptiste KE, Catry B, van Duijkeren E, Greko C, Moreno MA, et al. Macrolides and lincosamides in cattle and pigs: Use and development of antimicrobial resistance. Veterinary Journal. 2014;**200**:230-239. DOI: 10.1016/j.tvjl.2014.02.028

[62] Nobile CGA, Costantino R, Bianco A, Pileggi C, Pavia M. Prevalence and pattern of antibiotic resistance of *Campylobacter* spp. in poultry meat in Southern Italy. Food Control. 2013;**32**:715-718. DOI: 10.1016/j.foodcont.2013.02.011

[63] Kurinčič M, Botteldoorn N, Herman L, Smole MS. Mechanisms of erythromycin resistance of *Campylobacter* spp. isolated from food, animals and humans. International Journal of Food Microbiology. 2007;**120**:186-190. DOI: 10.1016/j.ijfoodmicro.2007.03.012

[64] Han F, Pu S, Wang F, Meng J, Ge B. Fitness cost of macrolide resistance in *Campylobacter jejuni*. International Journal of Antimicrobial Agents. 2009;**34**:462-466. DOI: 10.1016/j.ijantimicag.2009.06.019

[65] Wang Y, Zhang M, Deng F, Shen Z, Wu C, Zhang J, et al. Emergence of multidrug-resistant *Campylobacter* species isolates with a horizontally acquired rRNA methylase. Antimicrobial Agents and Chemotherapy. 2014;**58**:5405-5412. DOI: 10.1128/AAC.03039-14

[66] Kempf I, Kerouanton A, Bougeard S, Nagard B, Rose V, Mourand G, et al. *Campylobacter coli* in organic and conventional pig production in France and Sweden: Prevalence and antimicrobial resistance. Frontiers in Microbiology. 2017;**8**:955. DOI: 10.3389/fmicb.2017.00955

[67] Elhadidy M, Miller WG, Arguello H, Álvarez-Ordóñez A, Duarte A, Dierick K, et al. Genetic basis and clonal population structure of antibiotic resistance in *Campylobacter*

*jejuni* isolated from broiler carcasses in Belgium. Frontiers in Microbiology. 2018;**9**:1014. DOI: 10.3389/fmicb.2018.01014

[68] Fraqueza MJ, Ribeiro SA, Pereira SC, Fernandes MH, Fernandes MJ, Barreto AS. Genetic and antibiotic resistance profiles of thermophilic *Campylobacter* spp. isolated from quails (*Coturnix coturnix japonica*) in a Portuguese slaughterhouse. Food Control. 2016;**59**: 337-344. DOI: 10.1016/j.foodcont.2015.06.008

[69] Hoge CW, Gambel JM, Srijan A, Pitarangsi C, Echeverria P. Trends in antibiotic resistance among diarrheal pathogens isolated in Thailand over 15 years. Clinical Infectious Diseases. 1998;**26**:341-345. DOI: 10.1086/516303

[70] Luo N, Pereira S, Sahin O, Lin J, Huang S, Michel L, et al. Enhanced in vivo fitness of fluoroquinolone-resistant *Campylobacter jejuni* in the absence of antibiotic selection pressure. Proceedings of the National Academy of Sciences of the United States of America. 2005;**102**:541-546. DOI: 10.1073/pnas.0408966102

[71] Tribble DR. Resistant pathogens as causes of traveller's diarrhea globally and impact(s) on treatment failure and recommendations. Journal of Travel Medicine. 2017;**24**:S6-S12. DOI: 10.1093/jtm/taw090

[72] Zhang T, Dong J, Cheng Y, Lu Q, Luo Q, Wen G, et al. Genotypic diversity, antimicrobial resistance and biofilm-forming abilities of *Campylobacter* isolated from chicken in Central China. Gut Pathogens. 2017;**9**:62. DOI: 10.1186/s13099-017-0209-6

[73] Kurinčič M, Berce I, Zorman T, Smole MS. The prevalence of multiple antibiotic resistance in *Campylobacter* spp. from retail poultry meat. Food Technology and Biotechnology. 2005;**43**:157-163

[74] Kovač J, Čadež N, Stessl B, Stingl K, Gruntar I, Ocepek M, et al. High genetic similarity of ciprofloxacin-resistant *Campylobacter jejuni* in central Europe. Frontiers in Microbiology. 2015;**6**:1169. DOI: 10.3389/fmicb.2015.01169

[75] Kovaļenko K, Roasto M, Šantare S, Berziņš A, Hörman A. *Campylobacter* species and their antimicrobial resistance in Latvian broiler chicken production. Food Control. 2014;**46**: 86-90. DOI: 10.1016/j.foodcont.2014.05.009

[76] Lehtopolku M, Nakari UM, Kotilainen P, Huovinen P, Siitonen A, Hakanen AJ. Antimicrobial susceptibilities of multidrug-resistant *Campylobacter jejuni* and *C. coli* strains: In vitro activities of 20 antimicrobial agents. Antimicrobial Agents and Chemotherapy. 2010;**54**:1232-1236. DOI: 10.1128/AAC.00898-09

[77] Aguilar-Company J, Los-Arcos I, Pigrau C, Rodríguez-Pardo D, Larrosa MN, Rodríguez-Garrido V, et al. Potential use of fosfomycin-tromethamine for treatment of recurrent *Campylobacter* species enteritis. Antimicrobial Agents and Chemotherapy. 2016;**60**:4398-4400. DOI: 10.1128/AAC.00447-16

[78] Helms M, Simonsen J, Olsen KP, Molbak K. Adverse health events associated with antimicrobial drug resistance in *Campylobacter* Species: A registry-based cohort study. The Journal of Infectious Diseases. 2005;**191**:1050-1055. DOI: 10.1086/428453

[79] Iovine NM. Resistance mechanisms in *Campylobacter jejuni*. Virulence. 2013;**4**:230-240. DOI: 10.4161/viru.23753

[80] Kurinčič M, Klančnik A, Smole MS. Effects of efflux pump inhibitors on erythromycin, ciprofloxacin and tetracycline resistance in *Campylobacter* spp. isolates. Microbial Drug Resistance. 2012;**18**(5):492-501. DOI: 10.1089/mdr.2012.0017

[81] Mavri A, Smole MS. Resistance to bile salt and sodium deoxycholate in macrolide- and fluoroquinolone-susceptible and resistant *Campylobacter jejuni and Campylobacter coli* strains. Microbial Drug Resistance. 2013;**19**(3):168-174. DOI: 10.1089/mdr.2012.0217

[82] Kurinčič M, Klančnik A, Smole MS. Epigallocatechin gallate as a modulator of *Campylobacter* resistance to macrolide antibiotics. International Journal of Antimicrobial Agents. 2012;**40**:467-471. DOI: 10.1016/j.ijantimicag.2012.07.015

[83] Mavri A, Smole MS. Development of antimicrobial resistance in *Campylobacter jejuni* and *Campylobacter coli* adapted to biocides. International Journal of Food Microbiology. 2013;**160**:304-312. DOI: 10.1016/j.ijfoodmicro.2012.11.006

[84] Kovač J, Šimunović K, Wu Z, Klančnik A, Bucar F, Zhang Q, et al. Antibiotic resistance modulation and modes of action of (−)-α-Pinene in *Campylobacter jejuni*. PLoS One. 2015;**10**:1-14. DOI: 10.1371/journal.pone.0122871

[85] Ellington MJ, Ekelund O, Aarestrup FM, Canton R, Doumith M, Giske C, et al. The role of whole genome sequencing in antimicrobial susceptibility testing of bacteria: Report from the EUCAST Subcommittee. Clinical Microbiology and Infection. 2017;**23**:2-22. DOI: 10.1016/j.cmi.2016.11.012

[86] McDermott PF, Tyson GH, Kabera C, Chen Y, Li C, Folster JP, et al. Whole-genome sequencing for detecting antimicrobial resistance in nontyphoidal *Salmonella*. Antimicrobial Agents and Chemotherapy. 2016;**60**:5515-5520. DOI: 10.1128/AAC.01030-16

[87] Zankari E, Hasman H, Kaas RS, Seyfarth AM, Agersø Y, Lund O, et al. Genotyping using whole-genome sequencing is a realistic alternative to surveillance based on phenotypic antimicrobial susceptibility testing. The Journal of Antimicrobial Chemotherapy. 2013;**68**:771-777. DOI: 10.1093/jac/dks496

[88] Emond-Rheault JG, Jeukens J, Freschi L, Kukavica-Ibrulj I, Boyle B, Dupont MJ, et al. A Syst-OMICS approach to ensuring food safety and reducing the economic burden of salmonellosis. Frontiers in Microbiology. 2017;**8**:996. DOI: 10.3389/fmicb.2017.00996

[89] Whitehouse CA, Young S, Li C, Hsu CH, Martin G, Zhao S. Use of whole-genome sequencing for *Campylobacter* surveillance from NARMS retail poultry in the United States in 2015. Food Microbiology. 2018;**73**:122-128. DOI: 10.1016/j.fm.2018.01.018

[90] Leekitcharoenphon P, Garcia-Graells C, Botteldoorn N, Dierick K, Kempf I, Olkkola S, et al. Comparative genomics of quinolone-resistant and susceptible *Campylobacter jejuni* of poultry origin from major poultry producing European countries (GENCAMP). EFSA Supporting Publications. 2018. DOI: 10.2903/sp.efsa.2018.EN-1398

Chapter 3

# Antibiotic Use in Poultry Production and Its Effects on Bacterial Resistance

Christian Agyare, Vivian Etsiapa Boamah,
Crystal Ngofi Zumbi and Frank Boateng Osei

Additional information is available at the end of the chapter

http://dx.doi.org/10.5772/intechopen.79371

**Abstract**

A surge in the development and spread of antibiotic resistance has become a major cause for concern. Over the past few decades, no major new types of antibiotics have been produced and almost all known antibiotics are increasingly losing their activity against pathogenic microorganisms. The levels of multi-drug resistant bacteria have also increased. It is known that worldwide, more than 60% of all antibiotics that are produced find their use in animal production for both therapeutic and non-therapeutic purposes. The use of antimicrobial agents in animal husbandry has been linked to the development and spread of resistant bacteria. Poultry products are among the highest consumed products worldwide but a lot of essential antibiotics are employed during poultry production in several countries; threatening the safety of such products (through antimicrobial residues) and the increased possibility of development and spread of microbial resistance in poultry settings. This chapter documents some of the studies on antibiotic usage in poultry farming; with specific focus on some selected bacterial species, their economic importance to poultry farming and reports of resistances of isolated species from poultry settings (farms and poultry products) to essential antibiotics.

**Keywords:** bacteria, antibiotic resistance, antibiotics, antimicrobials, poultry

## 1. Introduction

Antibiotic resistance (AR) which is defined as the ability of an organism to resist the killing effects of an antibiotic to which it was normally susceptible [1] and it has become an issue of global interest [2]. This microbial resistance is not a new phenomenon since all microorganisms have an inherent capacity to resist some antibiotics [3]. However, the rapid surge in the development and spread of AR is the main cause for concern [4]. In recent years, enough evidence highlighting a link between excessive use of antimicrobial agents and antimicrobial resistance from animals as a contributing factor to the overall burden of AR has emerged [5]. The extent of usage is expected to increase markedly over coming years due to intensification of farming practices in most of the developing countries [6]. The main reasons for the use of antibiotics in food-producing animals include prevention of infections, treatment of infections, promotion of growth and improvement in production in the farm animals [7, 8].

Poultry is one of the most widespread food industries worldwide. Chicken is the most commonly farmed species, with over 90 billion tons of chicken meat produced per year [9]. A large diversity of antimicrobials, are used to raise poultry in most countries [10–12]. A large number of such antimicrobials are considered to be essential in human medicine [13, 14]. The indiscriminate use of such essential antimicrobials in animal production is likely to accelerate the development of AR in pathogens, as well as in commensal organisms. This would result in treatment failures, economic losses and could act as source of gene pool for transmission to humans. In addition, there are also human health concerns about the presence of antimicrobial residues in meat [15, 16], eggs [17] and other animal products [18, 19].

Generally, when an antibiotic is used in any setting, it eliminates the susceptible bacterial strains leaving behind those with traits that can resist the drug. These resistant bacteria then multiply and become the dominating population and as such, are able to transfer (both horizontally and vertically) the genes responsible for their resistance to other bacteria [1, 20]. Resistant bacteria can be transferred from poultry products to humans via consuming or handling meat contaminated with pathogens [21]. Once these pathogens are in the human system, they could colonize the intestines and the resistant genes could be shared or transferred to the endogenous intestinal flora, jeopardizing future treatments of infections caused by such organisms [5, 22–24].

## 2. Use of antibiotic in animal production

Antimicrobials' use in animal production dates as far back as the 1910 when due to shortage of meat products, workers carried out protests and riots across America [25]. Scientists at that time started looking for means of producing more meat at relatively cheaper costs; resulting in the use of antibiotics and other antimicrobial agents [26]. With the global threat of antibiotic resistance and increasing treatment failures, the non-therapeutic use of antibiotics in animal production has been banned in some countries [8, 27–29]. Sweden is known to be the first country to ban the use of antimicrobials for non-therapeutic purposes between 1986 (for growth promotion) and 1988 (for prophylaxis) [27]. This move was followed by Denmark, The Netherlands, United Kingdom and other European Union countries [27]. These countries also moved a step further and banned the use of all essential antibiotics as prophylactic agents in 2011 [30].

Several other countries have withdrawn the use of some classes of antibiotics or set up structures that regulate the use of selected antibiotics in animal production [29]. Despite these developments, it is currently estimated that over 60% of all antibiotics produced are used in livestock production, including poultry [6, 31].

The use of antibiotics in poultry and livestock production is favorable to farmers and the economy as well because it has generally improved poultry performance effectively and economically but at the same time, the likely dissemination of antibiotic resistant strains of pathogenic and non-pathogenic organisms into the environment and their further transmission to humans via the food chain could also lead to serious consequences on public health [32].

## 3. Antimicrobial resistance

Bacteria counteract the actions of antibiotics by four well-known mechanisms, namely; enzyme modification, alteration in target binding sites, efflux activity and decreased permeability of bacterial membrane [33]. This expression of resistance towards antibiotics by bacteria could either be intrinsic or acquired. Intrinsic resistance is due to inherent properties within the bacteria chromosome such as mutations in genes and chromosomally inducible enzyme production [34], whereas acquired resistance could be due to the transmission of resistance genes from the environment and/or horizontally transfer from other bacteria [35, 36].

## 4. Antibiotic resistance of some selected organisms in poultry

### 4.1. *Staphylococcus* species

The bacterial genus *Staphylococcus* is a Gram-positive cocci and a facultative anaerobe which appears in clusters when viewed under the microscope [37]. They are etiological agents of staphylococcosis, pododermatitis (bumblefoot) and septicaemia which affect mostly chicken and turkeys. Coagulase-negative species have also been implicated in human and animal infections [38, 39].

β-lactams were considered the first line of drugs for treatment of staphylococcal infections but due to emergence of high level of resistance to these and other drugs, there are currently very few drugs available for treatment of these infections [40]. Methicillin resistant *Staphylococcus aureus* (MRSA), now known as a superbug, is resistant to almost every available antibiotic used against *Staphylococcus* [41].

A study to detect the presence of MRSA in broilers, turkeys and the surrounding air in Germany reported the prevalence of MRSA in air as high as 77% in broilers compared to 54% in Turkeys. Ten different spa types were identified with spa type t011 and clonal complex (CC) 398 being the most prevalent. It was also found that for every farm, the same sequence types were present in both the birds and the environment [42]. This pattern of resistance was also reported in India with 1.6% of staphylococcal isolates containing mecA resistant gene [43].

In Africa, studies carried out in Ghana and Nigeria have shown that livestock-associated *Staphylococci* are susceptible to amoxicillin/clavulanic acid, amikacin, ciprofloxacin, gentamycin and cephalexin [39, 44], whereas in the US, most of the staphylococcal isolates were susceptible to rifampin, cotrimoxazole, gentamycin, vancomycin and chloramphenicol [45, 46]. It is worth noting that most of these organisms showed a high level of resistance to oxacillin and tetracycline, which would be disastrous if these oxacillin-resistant strains are transferred to humans [39, 44, 45].

### 4.2. *Pseudomonas* species

*Pseudomonas* is a genus of Gram-negative, aerobic bacteria that belongs to the family Pseudomonadaceae [47]. The genus *Pseudomonas* is ubiquitous in soil, water and on plants. It consists of 191 subspecies belonging to species groups including *P. fluorescens, P. pertucinogena, P. aeruginosa, P. chlororaphis, P. putida, P. stutzeri* and *P. syringae*. Pseudomoniasis, which is an opportunistic *P. aeruginosa* infection, is common in poultry birds like chickens, turkeys, ducks, geese and ostriches where infections in eggs destroy embryos [48].

*P. aeruginosa* causes respiratory infection, sinusitis, keratitis/keratoconjuctivitis and septicemia and responsible for pyogenic infections, septicemia, endocarditis and lameness along with many diverse diseases [49]. Infections may occur through skin wounds, contaminated vaccines and antibiotic solutions or needles used for injection. The disease may be systemic, affecting multiple organs and tissues or localized in tissues as infraorbital sinus or air sacs producing swelling of the head, wattles, sinuses and joints in poultry birds. *P. aeruginosa* has been isolated from many poultry farms and birds worldwide [49].

A study carried out in Ghana show that *P. aeruginosa* isolated from poultry litter were all susceptible to levofloxacin in the range of 20–100% and nearly 75% demonstrated intermediate susceptibility to aztreonam. The organisms showed resistance to cephalosporins, carbapenems, penicillins, quinolones, monobactam and aminoglycoside. Metallo β-Lactamase encoding genes (blaIMP, blaVIM) were not detected in any of the isolates but the class 1 integron which is known to carry multiple antibiotic resistant genes were detected in 89.4% of the multi-drug resistant strains [50]. This is contrary to a report by Zhang and his Colleagues [51], who identified the blaVIM gene in *P. aeruginosa* and *P. putida* from chicken that resembled corresponding regions in clinical isolates of *P. aeruginosa*. These isolates were resistant to all β-lactam antibiotics tested, including meropenem, imipenem, aztreonam, and ceftazidime [33, 51].

Another study in Nigeria reported that the *P. aeruginosa* isolates were highly resistant to β-lactams, tetracycline, tobramycin, nitrofurantoin and sulfamethoxazole-trimethoprim, while ofloxacin, imipenem and ertapenem were highly effective against the bacterial pathogens [52].

In Pakistan, a study which investigated the causative agents for necropsy in chicken, recorded a 28% prevalence for *P. aeruginosa*. These isolates were found to be 100% resistant towards ceftriaxone, meropenem, ciprofloxacin, erythromycin and colistin, while 60% sensitivity was observed against ampicillin sulbactam, ceftazidime, cefoperazone and rifampicin. Isolates exhibited variable multidrug resistance patterns to other antibiotics [53].

### 4.3. *Escherichia* species

*Escherichia coli* is a Gram-negative bacterium that has been known for ages to easily and frequently exchange genetic information through horizontal gene transfer with other related bacteria. Hence, it may exhibit characteristics based on the source of isolation. *E. coli* is a commensal organism living in the intestines of both humans and animals. However, some strains have been reported to cause gastrointestinal illnesses [54]. Tetracycline which is commonly used in poultry has been reported to be one of the drugs bacteria are most resistant to. There is a reported tetracycline resistance in poultry even without the administration of this antibiotic [21].

A study carried out on fecal isolates of *E. coli* in the Netherlands showed that there is a high level of multidrug resistance occurring in broilers, turkeys while majority of those from laying hens were susceptible. It was observed that the isolates from birds had high rates of resistance to amoxycillin alone and others had resistance to amoxicillin as well as oxytetracycline, streptomycin, sulfamethoxazole and trimethoprim. [55].

*E. coli* had a prevalence of 46.98% among the other bacteria isolated in Ghana. All isolates showed some degree of resistance to ceftriaxone (1.34%), cefotaxime (0.67%), gentamycin (2.01%), cotrimoxazole (1.34%), tetracycline (2.01%) and ampicillin (3.36%) [56]. Resistant genes have been found in *E. coli* isolates from Nigeria and these include bla-TEM (85%), sul2 (67%), sul3 (17%), aadA (65%), strA (70%), strB (61%), catA1 (25%), cmlA1 (13%), tetA (21%) and tetB (17%) which conveyed resistance to the following antibiotics; tetracycline (81%), sulfamethoxazole (67%), streptomycin (56%), trimethoprim (47%), ciprofloxacin (42%), ampicillin (36%), spectinomycin (28%), nalidixic acid (25%), chloramphenicol (22%), neomycin (14%) gentamicin (8%). In this study the isolates were susceptible to amoxicillin-clavulanate, ceftiofur, cefotaxime, colistin, florfenicol and apramycin. Class 1 and 2 integrons were found in five (14%) and six (17%) isolates, respectively, while one isolate contained both classes of integrons. There is that suggestion that poultry production environments represent important reservoirs of antibiotic resistance genes such as qnrS that may spread from livestock production farms to human populations via manure and water [57].

### 4.4. *Salmonella* species

*Salmonella* spp. are Gram-negative, facultative anaerobic, non-spore forming, usually motile rods belonging to the Enterobacteriaceae family, which are found in the alimentary tract of animals [37, 58]. Fecal shedding allows *Salmonella* to be transmitted among birds in a flock. *Salmonella* spp. is widespread in poultry production. Prevalence varies considerably depending on country and type of production as well as the detection methods applied. It is known to be the etiological agent responsible for salmonellosis by *Salmonella* spp. in both humans and animals. Food-borne salmonellosis caused still occurs throughout the world [58]. The risk factors associated with *Salmonella* infections and contamination in broiler chickens include contaminated chicks, size of the farm and contaminated feed and these risk increase when feed trucks are parked near the entrance of the workers' change room and when chicken are fed with meals [59, 60]. It also depends on age of the chicken, animal health, survival of organism in the gastric barrier, diet and genetic constitution of the chicken could also affect the colonization ability of *Salmonella* spp. in poultry [61].

Pullorum disease in poultry is caused by the *S. pullorum*. Transmission of the disease in birds can be vertical (transovarian) but also occurs through direct or indirect contact with infected birds via respiratory route or fecal matter or contaminated feed, water, or litter. Antimicrobials used to treat pullorum disease are furazolidone, gentamycin sulfate and antimetabolites (sulfadimethoxine, sulfamethazine and sulfamerazine) [62].

*Salmonella* spp. have increasingly been isolated from poultry with prevalence of 2.7% in Brazil and the most common isolates were *Salmonella enteritidis* (48.8%), *S. infantis* (7.6%), *S. typhimurium* (7.2%), and *S. heidelberg* (6.4%). All the isolated strains were resistant to at least one class of antimicrobial and 53.2% showed multidrug resistance to three or more classes, with streptomycin (89.2%), sulfonamides (72.4%), florfenicol (59.2%), and ampicillin (44.8%) [63].

*Salmonella* spp. are one of the commonest microbial contaminants in the poultry industry. In Ghana, there is high prevalence rate of 44.0% in poultry with main isolates being *S. kentucky* (18.1%), *S. nima* (12.8%), *S. muenster* (10.6%), *S. enteritidis* (10.6%) and *S. virchow* (9.6%). Resistance of these isolates to the various antibiotics were nalidixic acid (89.5%), tetracycline (80.7%), ciprofloxacin (64.9%), sulfamethazole (42.1%), trimethoprim (29.8%) and ampicillin (26.3%).

### 4.5. *Streptococcus* species

Streptococcus is Gram-positive bacteria. *Streptococcus gallolyticus* is a common member of the gut microbiota in animals and humans; however, being a zoonotic agent, it has been reported to cause mastitis in cattle, septicemia in pigeons, and meningitis, septicemia, and endocarditis in humans [64]. A study carried out in Japan isolated *Streptococcus gallolyticus* from pigeons with septicaemia. Most of the isolates were susceptible to vancomycin, penicillin G and ampicillin, while some were resistant to tetracycline, doxycycline and lincomycin. All the isolates were resistant to tetracycline had tet(M) and/or tet(L) and/or tet(O) genes [65].

### 4.6. *Campylobacter* species

*Campylobacter jejuni* and *Campylobacter coli* are the most prevalent disease causing species of the genus *Campylobacter*. They are mostly responsible for foodborne gastroenteritis in humans [66–68]. Campylobacteriosis is often associated with handling of raw poultry or eating of undercooked poultry meat [69]. Cross-contamination of raw poultry to other ready-to-eat foods via the cook's hands or kitchen utensils has been reported. Erythromycin is usually the drug of choice for the treatment of *Campylobacter* infections [68]. However, fluoroquinolones, gentamicin, and tetracycline are also clinically effective in treating *Campylobacter* infections when antimicrobial therapy is required [70].

Resistance of *C. jejuni* and *C. coli* isolates to fluoroquinolones, tetracycline, and erythromycin has been reported. The increased resistance is partly due to the wide use of these antimicrobials in animal husbandary, especially in poultry [71, 72].

A study carried out by Elz'bieta and his colleagues, in their quest to compare the prevalence and genetic background of antimicrobial resistance in Polish strains of *C. jejuni* and *C. coli* isolated from chicken carcasses and children reported a slight difference in resistance between human and chicken strains. The isolated *Campylobacter* strains were found to be resistant to gentamycin, tetracycline, ampicillin, ciprofloxacin and erythromycin and *tet(O)* gene and mutations in the *gyrA* genes were found to be associated with the observed antibiotic resistance in the study [73].

Another study carried out in Kenya isolated thermophilic *Campylobacter* species (*C. jejuni* and *C. coli*) from feces and clocal swabs of chicken. These isolates showed a high rate of resistance to nalidixic acid, tetracycline and ciprofloxacin of 77.4, 71.0 and 71.0%, respectively. Low resistance (25.8%) was detected for gentamicin and chloramphenicol and 61.3% of *C. jejuni* isolates exhibited multidrug resistance and 54.5% of the *C. jejuni* isolates possessed the *tet(O)* gene whereas all of *C. coli* had the *tet(A)* gene [74].

*C. jejuni* and *C. coli* are the predominant species of *Campylobacter* usually isolated from poultry farms. In Ghana, other species such as *Campylobacter lari*, *Campylobacter hyo-intestinalis* and *C. jejuni sub sp. doylei* have been isolated from poultry. These organisms have been found to be resistant to β-lactams, quinolones, aminoglycosides, erythromycin, tetracycline, chloramphenicol and trimethoprim-sulfamethoxazole and all isolated species were sensitive to imipenem [75, 76].

### 4.7. *Yersinia* species

It is a Gram-negative non-spore-forming rod, a psychrotrophic bacterium and able to survive and multiply at cold temperatures. Poultry meat is one of the most important sources of *Yersinia* spp. infections in humans. *Yersinia enterocolitica* is the predominant specie mostly isolated from poultry and poultry products [77]. In humans, *Y. enterocolitica* is an enteric pathogen which commonly causes acute enteritis associated with fever, bloody diarrhea and inflammation of lymph nodes. Contaminated food is one of the main sources of yersiniosis in humans [77].

*Y. enterocolitica* is widely distributed in nature and animals; food and environment are routinely contaminated with this organism. Major reservoir of *Y. enterocolitica* is swine. However, *Y. enterocolitica* has been frequently isolated from poultry and ready-to-eat foods [78]. A study in Iran reported a prevalence rate of *Y. enterocolitica* of 30% of among chicken meat samples [79]. *Yersinia* isolates (16%) from chicken and beef meat samples were mostly resistant to cephalotin (98%) and ampicillin (52%) [80].

*Y. enterocolitica* isolated from poultry raw meat and retailed meats in Poland were classified as biotype 1A and exhibited moderate ability of producing biofilms and ystB was the predominant virulence gene. In biofilms, a multi-system that include poor antibiotic penetration, nutrient limitation and slow growth, adaptive stress responses, and formation of persister cells are hypothesized to constitute the organisms' resistance to antibiotics [81].

### 4.8. *Clostridium* species

*Clostridium* is a genus of Gram-positive obligate anaerobic bacteria which includes several significant human pathogens. Spore of *Clostridium* normally inhabits soil and intestinal tract of animals and humans [82]. Common infections caused by *Clostridia* include botulism caused by *C. botulinum*, pseudomembranous colitis caused by *C. difficile*, cellulitis and gas gangrene caused by *C. perfringens*, tetanus caused by *C. tetani* and fatal post-abortion infections caused by *C. sordellii* [83].

High-dose penicillin-G remains sensitive to *Clostridia* species and thus widely used to treat Clostridial infections. *Clostridia* species such as *welchii* and tetani respond to sulfonamides [82]. Tetracyclines, carbapenems, metronidazole, vancomycin and chloramphenicol are effective options for treatment of *Clostridia* infections [84].

*C. perfringens* is known to cause necrotic enteritis in poultry. Bacitracin or virginiamycin is an effective treatment option when administered in the feed or drinking water. *C. colinum* is responsible for ulcerative enteritis. Bacitracin and penicillins are the most effective drugs in the treatment and prevention of this infection [85, 86].

A study in Egypt, identified 125 isolates of *C. perfringens* from clinical cases of necrotic enteritis in broiler chickens from 35 chicken coops and the all isolates were resistant to gentamycin, streptomycin, oxolinic acid, lincomycin, erythromycin and spiramycin. Over 95% of isolates were resistant to sulfamethoxazole-trimethoprim, doxycycline, perfloxacin, colistin and neomycin. Most of the isolates were susceptible to amoxicillin, ampicillin, fosfomycin, florfenicol and cephradine [85].

Thirty strains of *C. perfringens* isolated from chickens with necrotic enteritis in Korea were found to susceptible to ampicillin, amoxicillin/clavulanic acid, cephalothin, cefepime, chloramphenicol, cefoxitin, ceftiofur, florfenicol and penicillin but resistant to gentamycin, neomycin, streptomycin, apramycin and colistin [87]. This trend of resistance was similar to that observed in 43 *C. perfringens* isolates from the ileum of 5-week old broiler chicken in Taiwan. Most of the *C. perfringens* isolates were susceptible to amoxicillin, bacitracin and enrofloxacin but resistant to erythromycin, lincomycin and chlortetracycline [88].

### 4.9. *Bacillus* species

*Bacillus* is a genus of Gram-positive, obligate aerobic or facultative anaerobic rod shaped bacteria of the phylum firmicutes. *Bacillus* spp. include both free-living non-parasitic and parasitic pathogenic species [89]. Medically significant species include *B. anthracis* which causes anthrax and *B. cereus* which causes food poisoning [90]. Other infections caused by *Bacilli* spp. include pneumonia, endocarditis, ocular and musculoskeletal infections. Antibiotics usually used for *Bacillus* infections include vancomycin, imipenem, ciprofloxacin, gentamycin, tetracycline, chloramphenicol, clindamycin and erythromycin. Most *Bacillus* spp. have been found to be resistant to broad spectrum cephalosporins and ticarcillin-clavulanate [91].

In a study involving 18 strains of *B. cereus* isolated from raw and processed poultry meat from supermarkets in Iasi county, all the isolates were found to be resistant to penicillin, amoxicillin, amoxicillin-clavulanate, colistin, cefoperazone, sulfamethizole and metronidazole but sensitive to erythromycin, cotrimoxazole, tylosin, flumequine, kanamycin, gentamycin, enrofloxacin, oxolinic acid, apramycin, tetracycline and doxacilin. All *B. cereus* isolates were resistant to nearly half of tested antibiotics [92]. This pattern of resistance was also observed in 44 strains of *B. cereus* isolated from chicken and chicken products in the Jammu region of India. All isolates were resistant to penicillin G but sensitive to streptomycin. Over 60% of isolates were resistant to amoxicillin, ampicillin and carbenicillin [93].

### 4.10. *Mycobacterium* species

*Mycobacteria* are acid-fast, aerobic, nonmotile of bacteria of the genus *Mycobacterium* [94]. *Mycobacteria* are widespread organisms that live in water and food sources and can colonize their hosts without showing any adverse signs and symptoms. Pathogenic mycobacterial species including *M. tuberculosis, M. bovis, M. africanum, M. macroti* cause tuberculosis whiles *M. leprae* is responsible for leprosy. *Mycobacteria* spp. are naturally resistant to penicillin and mostly susceptible to clarithromycin and rifamycin [95].

A study in Bangladesh identified three *Mycobacterium* isolates from 80 poultry droppings and all isolates were found to be resistant to rifampicin but highly susceptible to azithromycin, ciprofloxacin, streptomycin and doxycycline. One isolate was identified as multi-drug resistant [96].

### 4.11. *Klebsiella* species

*Klebsiella* is a genus of non-motile, Gram-negative, oxidase-negative, rod-shaped bacteria with a prominent polysaccharide capsule and belong to the family *Enterobacteriaceae* [97]. *Klebsiella* species are found everywhere in nature including soil, plants, insect, humans and other animals [98]. Infections caused by *Klebsiella* spp. include septicaemia, meningitis, urinary tract infections, pneumonia, diarrhea [97]. Common pathogenic *Klebsiella* in humans and animals include *K. pneumoniae, K. oxytoca* and *K. variicola* [99]. Antibiotics commonly used in the treatment of *Klebsiella* infections include third-generation cephalosporins, carbapenems, aminoglycosides and quinolones [100].

A study in Langa, South Africa identified 102 sub-species of *K. pneumonia* (96 *K. ozaenae* and 6 *K. rhinoscleromatis* strains) from 17 free-range chicken samples. The isolates exhibited high level of resistance towards ampicillin (66.7%), nalidixic acid (61.8%), tetracycline (59.8%) and trimethoprim (50.0%) but highly susceptible towards gentamycin (3.9%) and ciprofloxacin (4.8%). Almost 40% of the isolates were found to be multi-drug resistant *K. pneumonia* strains [99]. Similar trend of resistance was observed among 77 *K. pneumoniae* isolates from poultry birds in Ekiti-state, Nigeria. The isolates showed high level of resistance towards tetracycline (100%), amoxicillin (94.8%), cotrimoxazole (94.8%) and augmentin (85.7%) [98].

### 4.12. *Enterococcus* species

*Enterococcus* is a large genus of Gram-positive diplococci, lactic acid-producing bacteria of the phylum Firmicutes [101]. Commonly found species include *Enterococcus faecalis* and *Enterococcus faecium* [102]. Notable infections caused by *Enterococci* include urinary tract infections, bacteremia, meningitis, endocarditis [103]. Antibiotics active against *Enterococci* include ampicillin, penicillin, nitrofurantoin and vancomycin [104]. *Enterococci* often possess intrinsic resistance towards β-lactam antibiotics and aminoglycosides. However, resistance of *Enterococci* to vancomycin has been reported in several studies [105–107].

A study in Czech Republic identified 228 enterococcal isolates from the intestinal tract of poultry. These isolates were found to be highly resistant to tetracycline (80%), erythromycin (59%) and ofloxacin (51%) but exhibited low resistance to ampicillin (3%) and ampicillin/sulbactam (3%) [105]. A similar trend of resistance was reported among 163 Enterococcal isolates from poultry litter in the Abbotsford area of British Columbia, Canada. The identified enterococcal isolates were found to be highly resistant to lincomycin (80.3%), tetracycline (65.3%), penicillin (61.1%) but showed low resistance towards to nitrofurantoin (3.8%), daptomycin (3.5%) and gentamycin (0.8%) [108]. There is a high possibility of multi-drug resistant enterococci in animal meat and fecal matter being transferred to humans [106].

### 4.13. *Proteus* species

*Proteus* is a genus of Gram-negative Proteobacteria which is widely distributed as saprophytes [109]. They are mainly found in decomposing animal matter, sewage, manure, mammalian intestine, human and animal fecal matter. They are mainly opportunistic pathogens responsible for nosocomial urinary and septic infections [110]. Three species, namely, *P. vulgaris, P. mirabilis* and *P. penneri* are the only opportunistic species responsible for human infections. Most strains of *P. mirabilis* are sensitive to ampicillin and cephalosporins whereas *P. vulgaris* strains are not sensitive to these antibiotics [109].

A study in Iran identified 54 *P. mirabilis* isolates from chicken intestines and 54 *P. mirabilis* isolates were screened for antimicrobial susceptibility to 13 antimicrobial agents. None of the *P. mirabilis* isolates in this study were found to be resistant to gentamycin. Over 90% of isolates were resistant to nalidixic acid, doxycycline and tetracycline. Less than a quarter of isolates were resistant to norfloxacin, ampicillin, amikacin and ceftriaxone. Nearly 96% of the isolates were resistant to at least two or more antibiotics. One isolate exhibited resistance to 10 antibiotics whereas three and five isolates were resistant to nine and seven antibiotics, respectively. The results showed that chicken could be a source of antibiotic resistant and multi-drug resistant *P. mirabilis* strains and these resistant strains can cause worldwide problem both for veterinary sector and public health [111].

A similar trend of antibiotic resistance was observed in 36 *P. mirabilis* isolates from chicken droppings from commercial poultry farms in Bangladesh. Nearly 95% of the isolates were resistant to tetracycline followed by nalidixic acid (89%) and almost 20% of the isolates were found to be resistant to ciprofloxacin and 84% of the isolates exhibited multidrug resistance [112].

## 5. Other species of importance

Infections from other bacterial species could also result in the use of antibiotics. These include Mycoplasmosis (caused by *Mycoplasma gallisepticum, Mycoplasma meleagridis* and *Mycoplasma synoviae*) [86], *Pasteurella multocida* and *Haemophilus gallinarum* infections [62, 113]. These infections usually require the use broad spectrum antibiotics including tylosin, aureomycin, terramycin, gallimycin, penicillin, erythromycin, sulfadimethoxine, sulfathiazole and other sulfa drugs administered either in the feed, drinking water or by injections [62].

## 6. Conclusion

Several bacterial species are the major causes of infections in poultry and other animal husbandry. Most of these infections are linked to foodborne outbreaks, live animal contact, poor hygiene, and environmental exposure. With the emergence of antimicrobial resistance, the pathogenicity and virulence of these organisms have increased and treatment options are diminishing and also more expensive. Multidrug resistant bacteria have been found in poultry, poultry products, carcasses, litter and fecal matter of birds and these pose a risk to both handlers, consumers and a threat to global and public health. The above information also calls for increased surveillance measures and monitoring of antibiotic usage in both animal husbandry and humans throughout the world.

## Author details

Christian Agyare*, Vivian Etsiapa Boamah, Crystal Ngofi Zumbi and Frank Boateng Osei

*Address all correspondence to: cagyare.pharm@knust.edu.gh

Department of Pharmaceutics, Faculty of Pharmacy and Pharmaceutical Sciences, Kwame Nkrumah University of Science and Technology, Kumasi, Ghana

## References

[1] Madigan MT, Martinko JM, Bender KS, Buckley FH, Stahl DA. Brock Biology of Microorganisms. 14th ed. Illinois: Pearson International; 2014. p. 1006

[2] Antimicrobial Resistance Global Report on Surveillance. Geneva: World Health Organization; 2014: 256. Retrieved from: http://www.who.int/drugresistance/documents/surveillancereport/en/ on 15th April, 2018

[3] Hugo WB, Russel AD. Pharmaceutical Microbiology. 6th ed. Oxford: Blackwell Science Ltd; 1998. p. 514

[4] Aarestrup FM, Wegener HC, Collignon P. Resistance in bacteria of the food chain: Epidemiology and control strategies. Expert Review of Anti-Infective Therapy. 2008;**6**: 733-750

[5] Marshall BM, Levy SB. Food animals and antimicrobials: Impacts on human health. Clinical Microbiology Reviews. 2011;**24**:718-733

[6] Van Boeckel TP, Brower C, Gilbert M, Grenfell BT, Levin SA, Robinson TP, Teillant A, Laxminarayan R. Global trends in antimicrobial use in food animals. Proceedings of the National Academy of Sciences. 2015;**112**:5649-5654

[7] Mathew AG, Liamthong S, Lin J. Evidence of Int 1 transfer between *Escherichia coli* and *Salmonella typhi*. Food Biology. 2009;**6**(8):959-964

[8] Castanon JIR. History of the use of antibiotic as growth promoters in European poultry feeds. Poultry Science. 2007;**86**:2466-2471

[9] Food and Agricultural Organization. FAO Publications Catalogue 2017. United Nations: Food and Agricultural Organization; 2017. Retrieved from http://www.fao.org/3/b-i6407e.pdf on 14th April, 2018

[10] Landers TF, Cohen B, Wittum TE, Larson EL. A review of antibiotic use in food animals: Perspective, policy, and potential. Public Health Reports. 2012;**127**(1):4-22

[11] Sahoo KC, Tamhankar AJ, Johansson E, Lundborg CS. Antibiotic use, resistance development and environmental factors: A qualitative study among healthcare professionals in Orissa, India. BioMedical Central Public Health. 2010;**10**:629

[12] Boamah VE, Agyare C, Odoi H, Dalsgaard A. Antibiotic practices and factors influencing the use of antibiotics in selected poultry farms in Ghana. Journal of Antimicrobial Agents. 2016;**2**:120. DOI: 10.4172/2472-1212.1000120

[13] World Health Organization Model List of Essential Medicines. Geneva: World Health Organization; 2010:1-43. Retrieved from http://www.who.int/medicines/publications/essentialmedicines/en/ on 13th April, 2018

[14] World Health Statistics 2017: Monitoring Health for the Sustainable Development Goals. Geneva: World Health Organization; 2017. Retrieved from http://apps.searo.who.int/PDS_DOCS/B5348.pdf on the 10th April, 2018

[15] Mirlohi M, Aalipour F, Jalali M. Prevalence of antibiotic residues in commercial milk and its variation by season and thermal processing methods. International Journal of Environmental Health Engineering. 2013;**2**:41

[16] Darwish WS, Eldaly EA, El-Abbasy MT, Ikenaka Y, Nakayama S, Ishizuka M. Antibiotic residues in food: The African scenario. Japanese Journal of Veterinary Research. 2013; **61**:S13-S22

[17] Goetting V, Lee KA, Tell LA. Pharmacokinetics of veterinary drugs in laying hens and residues in eggs: A review of the literature. Journal of Veterinary Pharmacology and Therapy. 2011;**34**:521-556

[18] Addo KK, Mensah GI, Aning KG, Nartey N, Nipah GK, Bonsu C, Akyeh ML, Smits HL. Microbiological quality and antibiotic residues in informally marketed raw cow milk within the coastal savannah zone of Ghana. Tropical Medicine and International Health. 2011;**16**:227-232

[19] Mehdizadeh S, Kazerani HR, Jamshidi A. Screening of chloramphenicol residues in broiler chickens slaughtered in an industrial poultry abattoir in Mashhad, Iran. Iranian Journal of Veterinary Science and Technology. 2010;**2**:25-32

[20] Laxminarayan R, Duse A, Wattal C, Zaidi AKM, Wertheim HFL, Sumpradit N, Vlieghe E, Hara GL, Gould IM, Goossens H, Greko C, So AD, Bigdeli M, Tomson G, Woodhouse W, Ombaka E, Peralta AQ, Qamar FN, Mir F, Kariuki S, Bhutta ZA, Coates A, Bergstrom R, Wright GD, Brown ED, Cars O. Antibiotic resistance–The need for global solutions. Lancet Infectious Diseases. 2013;**13**:1057-1098

[21] van, den Bogaard AE, Stobberingh EE. Epidemiology of resistance to antibiotics: Links between animals and humans. International Journal of Antimicroial. Agents. 2000;**14**: 327-335

[22] Hall MAL, Dierikx CM, Stuart JC, Voets GM, van den Munckhof MP. Dutch patients, retail chicken meat and poultry share the same ESBL genes, plasmids and strains. Clinical Microbiology and Infection. 2011;**17**(6):873-880

[23] Jakobsen L, Kurbasic A, Skjøt-rasmussen L, Ejrnæs K, Porsbo LJ, Pedersen K, Jensen LB, Emborg H, Agersø Y, Olsen KEP, Aarestrup FM, Frimodt-møller N, Hammerum AM. *Escherichia coli* isolates from broiler chicken meat, broiler chickens, pork and pigs share phylogroups and antimicrobial resistance with community-dwelling. Foodborne Pathogens and Disease. 2010;**7**:537-547

[24] de Leener E, Martel A, de Graef EM, Top J, Butaye P, Haesebrouck F, Willems R, Decostere A. Molecular analysis of human, porcine, and poultry *Enterococcus faecium* isolates and their erm (B) genes. Applied Environmental Microbiology. 2005;**71**:2766-2770

[25] Ogle M. In Meat We Trust: An Unexpected History of Carnivore America. New York: Houghton Mifflin Harcourt Publishing Company; 2013. p. 384

[26] Dibner JJ, Richards JD. Antibiotic growth promoters in agriculture: History and mode of action. Poultry Science. 2005;**84**:634-643

[27] Cogliani C, Goossens H, Greko C. Restricting antimicrobial use in food animals: Lessons from Europe. Microbe. 2011;**6**:274-279

[28] European Union. Ban on antibiotics as growth promoters in animal feed enters into effect. Regulation. Brussels: European Union. 2006. 1P:05:1687

[29] Choct M. Alternatives to in-feed antibiotics in monogastric animal industry. ASA Technical Bulletin. 2001;**30**:1-7

[30] Maron DF, Smith TJS, Nachman KE. Restrictions on antimicrobial use in food animal production: An international regulatory and economic survey. Globalization and Health. 2013;**9**:48

[31] van Boeckel TP, Gandra S, Ashok A, Caudron Q, Grenfell BT, Levin SA, Laxminarayan R. Global antibiotic consumption 2000 to 2010: An analysis of national pharmaceutical sales data. Lancet Infectious Diseases. 2014;**14**:742-750

[32] Apata DF. Antibiotic resistance in poultry. International Journal of Poultry Science. 2009;**8**:404-408

[33] Bassetti M, Merelli M, Temperoni C, Astilean A. New antibiotics for bad bugs: Where are. we? Annual Clinical Microbiology and Antimicrobials. 2013

[34] Davies J. Microbes have the last word. European Molecular Biology Organization Reports. 2007;**8**:616-621

[35] McDermott PF, Walker RD, White DG. Antimicrobials: Modes of action and mechanisms of resistance. International Journal of Toxicology. 2003;**22**:135-143

[36] Randall LP, Cooles SW, Osborn MK, Piddock LJV, Woodward MJ. Antibiotic resistance genes, integrons and multiple antibiotic resistance in thirty-five serotypes of *Salmonella*

*enterica* isolated from humans and animals in the UK. Journal of Antimicrobial Chemotherapy. 2004;**53**:208-216

[37] Barrow GI, Feltham RKA. Cowan and Steel's Manual for the Identification of Medical Bacteria. 3th ed. Cambridge, UK: Cambridge University Press; 2009. p. 331

[38] Koksal F, Yasar H, Samasti M. Antibiotic resistance patterns of coagulase-negative *Staphylococcus* strains isolated from blood cultures of septicemic patients in Turkey. Microbiology Research. 2009;**164**:404-410

[39] Boamah VE, Agyare C, Odoi H, Adu F, Gbedema S, Dalsgaard A. Prevalence and antibiotic resistance of coagulase-negative *Staphylococci* isolated from poultry farms in three regions of Ghana. Infection and Drug Resistance. 2017;**10**:175-183

[40] Mamza SA, Egwu GO, Mshelia GD. Beta-lactamase *Escherichia coli* and *Staphylococcus aureus* isolated from chickens in Nigeria. Veterinary Italian Journal. 2010;**46**:155-165

[41] Stapleton PD, Taylor PW. Methicillin resistance in *Staphylococcus aureus*. Science Progress. 2007;**85**:57-72

[42] Friese A, Schulz J, Zimmermann K, Tenhagen BA, Fetsch A, Hartung J, Rösler U. Occurrence of livestock-associated methicillin-resistant *Staphylococcus aureus* in Turkey and broiler barns and contamination of air and soil surfaces in their vicinity. Applied Environmental Microbiology. 2013;**79**:2759-2766

[43] Bhedi KR, Nayak JB, Brahmbhatt MN, Roy A. Detection and molecular characterization of methicillin-resistant *Staphylococcus aureus* obtained from poultry and poultry house environment of Anand district, Gujarat, India. International Journal Current Microbiology and Applied Sciences. 2018;**7**:867-872

[44] Suleiman A, Zaria LT, Grema HA, Ahmadu P. Antimicrobial resistant coagulase positive *Staphylococcus aureus* from chickens in Maiduguri, Nigeria. Sokoto Journal of Veterinary Science. 2013;**11**:51-55

[45] Waters AE, Contente-Cuomo T, Buchhagen J, Liu CM, Watson L, Pearce K, Foster JT, Bowers J, Driebe EM, Engelthaler DM, Keim PS, Price LB. Multidrug-resistant *Staphylococcus aureus* in US meat and poultry. Clinical Infectious Diseases. 2011;**52**:1227-1230

[46] Abdalrahman LS, Stanley A, Wells H, Fakhr MK. Isolation, virulence, and antimicrobial resistance of methicillin-resistant *Staphylococcus aureus* (MRSA) and methicillin sensitive *Staphylococcus aureus* (MSSA) strains from Oklahoma retail poultry meats. International Journal of Environmental Research and Public Health. 2015;**12**:6148-6161

[47] Skerman SV, McGowan V, Sneath P. Approved Lists of Bacterial Names (Amended). Approved List of Bacteria Names. Washington DC: ASM Press; 1989. p. 196

[48] de Vos P, Garrity GM, Jones D, Krieg NR, Ludwig W, Rainey FA, Schleifer KH, Whitman WB. Bergey's Manual of Systematic Bacteriology. New York: Springer: 2009. p. 1450

[49] Sams AR. Poultry Meat Processing. Boca Raton: CRC Press; 2001. p. 345

[50] Odoi H. Isolation and Characterization of Multi-Drug Resistant *Pseudomonas aeruginosa* from Clinical, Environmental and Poultry Litter Sources in Ashanti Region of Ghana (MPhil Thesis). Kumasi: Kwame Nkrumah University of Science and Technology; 2016

[51] Zhang R, Liu Z, Li J, Lei L, Yin W, Li M, Wu C, Walsh TR, Wang Y, Wang S, Wua Y. Presence of VIM-positive *Pseudomonas* species in chickens and their surrounding environment. Antimicrobial Agents and Chemotherapy. 2017;**61**:1-5

[52] Aniokette U, Iroha CS, Ajah MI, Nwakaeze AE. Occurrence of multi-drug resistant Gram-negative bacteria from poultry and poultry products sold in Abakaliki. Journal of Agricultural Science and Food Technology. 2016;**2**:119-124

[53] Sharma S, Galav V, Agrawal M, Faridi F, Kumar B. Multi-drug resistance pattern of bacterial flora obtained from necropsy samples of poultry. Journal of Animal Health and Production. 2017;**5**:165-171

[54] Tenaillon O, Skurnik D, Picard B, Denamur E. The population genetics of commensal *Escherichia coli*. National Review of Microbiology. 2010;**8**:207-217

[55] van den Bogaard AE, London N, Driessen C, Stobberingh EE. Antibiotic resistance of faecal *Escherichia coli* in poultry, poultry farmers and poultry slaughterers. Journal of Antimicrobial Chemotherapy. 2001;**47**(6):763-771

[56] Yao GM. Prevalence and Antibiotic Resistance of *Salmonella* sp., *Shigella* sp. and *Escherichia coli* in Fresh Retail Chicken in the Accra Metropolis. Accra: University of Ghana; 2015

[57] Adelowo OO, Fagade OE, Agersø Y. Antibiotic resistance and resistance genes in *Escherichia coli* from poultry farms, Southwest Nigeria. Journal of Infections in Developing Countries. 2014;**8**:1103-1112

[58] Bell C, Kyriakides A. *Salmonella*. A Practical Approach to the Organism and its Control in Foods. Oxford: Blackwell Science; 2007. p. 338

[59] Marin C, Balasch S, Vega S, Lainez M. Sources of *Salmonella* contamination during broiler production in eastern Spain. Preventive Veterinary Medicine. 2011;**98**:39-45

[60] Arsenault J, Letellier A, Quessy S, Normand V, Boulianne M. Prevalence and risk factors for *Salmonella* spp. and *Campylobacter* spp. faecal colonization in broiler chicken and Turkey flocks slaughtered in Quebec, Canada. Preventive Veterinary Medicine. 2007;**81**:250-264

[61] Cosby DE, Cox NA, Harrison MA, Wilson JL, Buhr RJ, Fedorka-Cray PJ. *Salmonella* and antimicrobial resistance in broilers: A review. Journal of Applied Poultry Research. 2015;**24**:408-426

[62] Msoffe PL, Aning KG, Byarugaba DK, Mbuthia PG, Sourou S, Cardona C, Bunn DA, Nyaga PN, Njagi LW, Maina AN, Kiama SG. Handbook of Poultry Diseases Important in Africa. CRSP: A Project of the Global Livestock; 2009. p. 83

[63] Medeiros MAN, de Oliveira DCN, Rodrigues DP, de Freitas DRC. Prevalence and antimicrobial resistance of *Salmonella* in chicken carcasses at retail in 15 Brazilian cities. Pan American Journal of Public Health. 2011;**30**:555-560

[64] de Herdt P, Devriese L, de Groote B, Ducatelle R, Haesebrouck F. Antibiotic treatment of *Streptococcus bovis* infections in pigeons. Avian Pathology. 1993;**22**:605-615

[65] Nomoto R, Tien LHT, Sekizaki T, Osawa R. Antimicrobial susceptibility of *Streptococcus gallolyticus* isolated from humans and animals. Japanese Journal of Infectious Diseases. 2013;**66**:334-336

[66] Sackey BA, Mensah P, Collison E, Sakyi-Dawson E. *Campylobacter, Salmonella, Shigella* and *Escherichia coli* in live and dressed poultry from Accra metropolitan. International Journal of Food Microbiology. 2001;**71**:21-28

[67] Wimalarathna HML, Richardson JF, Lawson AJ, Elson R, Meldrum R, Maiden MCJ, Mccarthy ND, Sheppard SK. Widespread Acquisition of Antimicrobial Resistance among *Campylobacter* Isolates from UK Retail Poultry and Evidence for Clonal Expansion of Resistant Lineages. BioMedical Central Microbiology; 2013

[68] Acheson D, Allos BM. *Campylobacter jejuni* infections: Update on emerging issues and trends. Clinical Infectious Diseases. 2001;**32**(8):1201-1206

[69] Altekruse SF, Stern NJ, Fields PI, Swerdlow DL. *Campylobacter jejuni*–An emerging foodborne pathogen. Emerging Infectious Diseases. 1999;**5**:28-35

[70] Moore JE, Deborah C, Dooley JSG, Fanning S, Lucey B, Matsuda M, Mcdowell DA, Mégraud FB, Millar C, O'Mahony R, O'Riordan L, O'Rourke M, Rao JR, Rooney PJ, Sails A, Whyte P. *Campylobacter*. Veterinary Research. 2005;**36**:351-382

[71] Wilson IG. Antibiotic resistance of *Campylobacter* in raw retail chickens and imported chicken portions. Epidemiology and Infection. 2003;**131**:1181-1186

[72] Randall LP, Ridley AM, Cooles SW, Sharma M, Sayers AR, Pumbwe L, Newell DG, Piddock LJV, Woodward MJ. Prevalence of multiple antibiotic resistance in 443 *Campylobacter* spp. isolated from humans and animals. Journal of Antimicrobial Chemotherapy. 2003;**52**:507-510

[73] Rożynek E, Dzierżanowska-Fangrat K, Korsak D, Konieczny P, Wardak S, Szych J, Jarosz M, Dzierżanowska D. Comparison of antimicrobial resistance of *Campylobacter jejuni* and *Campylobacter coli* isolated from humans and chicken carcasses in Poland. Journal of Food Protection. 2008;**71**:602-607

[74] Nguyen TNM, Hotzel H, Njeru J, Mwituria J, El-Adawy H, Tomaso H, Neubauer H, Hafez HM. Antimicrobial resistance of *Campylobacter* isolates from small scale and backyard chicken in Kenya. Gut Pathology. 2016;**8**:1-9

[75] Kumar VA, Steffy K, Chatterjee M, Sugumar M, Dinesh KR, Manoharan A, Karim S, Biswas R. Detection of oxacillin-susceptible mecA-positive *Staphylococcus aureus* isolates

by use of chromogenic medium MRSA ID. Journal of Clinical Microbiology. 2013; **51**(1):318-319

[76] Karikari AB, Obiri-Danso K, Frimpong EH, Krogfelt K.A. Antibiotic resistance of *Campylobacter* recovered from faeces and carcasses of healthy livestock. Biomed Research International. 2017; 4091856

[77] Annamalai T, Venkitanarayanan K. Expression of major cold shock proteins and genes by *Yersinia enterocolitica* in synthetic medium and foods. Journal of Food Protection. 2005;**68**:2454-2458

[78] Rahman A, Bonny TS, Stonsaovapak S, Ananchaipattana C. *Yersinia enterocolitica*: Epidemiological studies and outbreaks. Journal of Pathogens. 2011:1-11

[79] Sirghani K, Zeinali T, Jamshidi A. Detection of *Yersinia enterocolitica* in retail chicken meat, Mashhad, Iran. Journal of Pathogens. 2018;**2018**:1286216

[80] Dallal MMS, Doyle MP, Rezadehbashi M, Dabiri H, Sanaei M, Modarresi S, Bakhtiari R, Sharifiy K, Taremi M, Zali MR, Sharifi-Yazdi MK. Prevalence and antimicrobial resistance profiles of *Salmonella* serotypes, *Campylobacter* and *Yersinia* spp. isolated from retail chicken and beef, Tehran, Iran. Food Control. 2010;**21**(4):388-392

[81] Zadernowska A, Chaje W. Prevalence, bio film formation and virulence markers of *Salmonella* sp. and *Yersinia enterocolitica* in food of animal origin in Poland. LWT-Food Science and Technology. 2017;**75**:552-556

[82] Péchiné S, Collignon A. Immune responses induced by *Clostridium difficile*. Anaerobe. 2016;**41**:68-78

[83] Num SM, Useh NM. *Clostridium* : Pathogenic oles, industrial uses and medicinal prospects of natural products as ameliorative agents against pathogenic species. Jordan Journal of Biological Sciences. 2014;**7**(2):81-94

[84] Banawas SS. *Clostridium difficile* infections: A global overview of drug sensitivity and resistance mechanisms. Biomed Research International. 2018:1-9

[85] Osman KM, Elhariri M. Antibiotic resistance of *Clostridium perfringens* isolates from broiler chickens in Egypt. Review of Science and Technology. 2013;**32**(2):841-850

[86] Nhung NT, Chansiripornchai N, Carrique-Mas JJ. Antimicrobial resistance in bacterial poultry pathogens: A review. Frontiers in Veterinary Science. 2017;**4**:1-17

[87] Park JY, Kim S, Oh JY, Kim HR, Jang I, Lee HS, Kwon YK. Poultry science. 2015;**94**:1158-1164

[88] Fan YC, Wang CL, Wang C, Chen TC, Chou CH, Tsai HJ. Incidence and antimicrobial susceptibility to *Clostridium perfringens* in premarket broilers in Taiwan. Avian Disease. 2016;**60**(2):444-449

[89] Slepecky RA, Hemphill HE. The genus Bacillus-nonmedical. In: Balows A, Truper HG, Dworkin M, Harder W, Schleifer KH, editors. The Prokaryotes. 2nd ed. New York: Springer; 2009. p. 562

[90] Fagerlund A, Lindbäck T, Granum PE. *Bacillus cereus* cytotoxins Hbl, Nhe and CytK are secreted via the sec translocation pathway. BioMed Central Microbiology. 2012;**10**:304

[91] Reboli AC, Bryan CS, Farrar WE. Bacteremia and infection of a hip prosthesis caused by *Bacillus alvei*. Jounal of Clinical Microbiology. 1989;**27**(6):1395-1396

[92] Florişteán V, Cretu C, Carp-Cărare M. Bacteriological characteristics of *Bacillus Cereus* isolates from poultry. Bulletin of University of Agricultural Sciences and Veterinary Medicine Cluj-Napoca. 2007;**64**:1-2

[93] Bashir M, Malik MA, Javaid M, Badroo GA. Prevalence and characterization of *Bacillus cereus* in meat and meat products in and around Jammu region of Jammu and Kashmir, India. International Journal of Current Microbiology and Applied Sciences. 2017;**6**(12):1094-1106

[94] Rastogi N, Legrand E, Sola C. The mycobacteria: An introduction to nomenclature and pathogenesis. Review of Science Technology. 2001;**20**(1):21-54

[95] Barrow WW. Treatment of mycobacterial infections pathogenesis intracellular parasitism. Scientific and Technical Review of the Office International des Epizooties (Paris). 2001;**20**(1):55-70

[96] Reza M, Lijon M, Khatun M, Islam M. Prevalence and antibiogram profile of *Mycobacterium* spp. in poultry and its environments. Journal of Advanced Veterinary and Animal Research. 2015;**2**(4):458

[97] Podschun R, Ullmann U. *Klebsiella* spp. as nosocomial pathogens: Epidemiology, taxonomy, typing methods, and pathogenicity factors. Journal of Clinical Microbiology. 1998;**11**(4):589-603

[98] Ajayi AO, Egbebi AO. Antibiotic susceptibility of *Salmonella typhi* and *Klebsiella pneumoniae* from poultry and local birds in Ado-Ekiti, Ekiti-state. Nigeria. Annals of Biological Research. 2011;**2**(3):431-437

[99] Fielding BC, Mnabisa A, Gouws PA, Morris T. Antimicrobial-resistant *Klebsiella* species isolated from free-range chicken samples in an informal settlement. Archives of Medical Science. 2012;**8**(1):39-42

[100] van Duin D, Bonomo RA. Ceftazidime/avibactam and ceftolozane/tazobactam: Second-generation β-lactam/β-lactamase inhibitor combinations. Clinical Infectious Diseases. 2016;**63**(2):234-241

[101] Teixeira LM, De Janeiro R, Merquior VLC. Enterococcus. In: Filippis I, McKee M, editors. Molecular Typing in Bacterial Infections. New York: Springer Science; 2013. p. 17-27

[102] Gilmore MS, Clewell DB, Courvalin P. The Enterococci: Pathogenesis, Molecular Biology and Antibiotic Resistance. Washington, USA: ASM Press; 2002. p. 484

[103] Fisher K, Phillips C. The ecology, epidemiology and virulence of *Enterococcus*. Microbiology. 2009;**155**(6):1749-1757

[104] Zhanel GG, Laing NM, Nichol KA, Palatnick LP, Noreddin A, Hisanaga T, Johnson JL, Hoban DJ. Antibiotic activity against urinary tract infection (UTI) isolates of vancomycin-resistant *Enterococci* (VRE): Results from the 2002 north American vancomycin resistant *Enterococci* susceptibility study (NAVRESS). Journal of Antimicrobial Chemotherapy. 2003;**52**(3):382-388

[105] Kolář M, Pantůček R, Bardoň J, Vágnerová I, Typovská H, Válka I, Doškař J. Occurrence of antibiotic-resistant bacterial strains isolated in poultry. Veterinary Medicine (Praha). 2002;**47**(2-3):52-59

[106] Vignaroli C, Zandri G, Aquilanti L, Pasquaroli S, Biavasco F. Multidrug-resistant *enterococci* in animal meat and faeces and co-transfer of resistance from an *Enterococcus durans* to a human *Enterococcus faecium*. Current Microbiology. 2011;**62**(5):1438-1447

[107] Oguttu WJ. Antimicrobial Drug Resistance of Enteric Bacteria from Broilers Fed Antimicrobial Growth Enhancers and Exposed Poultry Abattior Workers [Thesis]. Pretoria: University of Pretoria; 2007

[108] Furtula V, Jackson CR, Farrell EG, Barrett JB, Hiott LM, Chambers PA. Antimicrobial resistance in *Enterococcus* spp. isolated from environmental samples in an area of intensive poultry production. International Journal of Environmental Research and Public Health. 2013;**10**(3):1020-1036

[109] Różalski A, Torzewska A, Moryl M, Kwil I, Maszewska A, Ostrowska K, Drzewiecka D, Zabłotni A, Palusiak A, Siwińska M, Stączek P. Proteus spp. – An opportunistic bacterial pathogen–Classification, swarming growth, clinical significance and virulence factors. Folia Biologica et Oecologica. 2012;**8**(1):1-17

[110] Ahmed DA. Prevalence of Proteus spp. in some hospitals in Baghdad City. Iraqi Journal of Science. 2015;**56**(1):665-672

[111] Nemati M. Antimicrobial resistance of *Proteus* isolates from poultry. European Journal of Experimental Biology. 2013;**3**(6):499-500

[112] Nahar A, Siddiquee M, Nahar S, Anwar KS, Ali SI, Islam S. Multidrug resistant-*Proteus mirabilis* isolated from chicken droppings in commercial poultry farms : Bio-security concern and emerging public health threat in Bangladesh. Biosafety and Health Education. 2014;**2**(2):120-125

[113] McEwen SA, Fedorka-Cray PJ. Antimicrobial use and resistance in animals. Clinical Infectious Diseases. 2002;**34**(3):S93-S106

Chapter 4

# Antibiotic Resistance in Lactic Acid Bacteria

Yenizey M. Álvarez-Cisneros and
Edith Ponce-Alquicira

Additional information is available at the end of the chapter

http://dx.doi.org/10.5772/intechopen.80624

**Abstract**

Most starter cultures belong to the lactic acid bacteria group (LAB) and recognized as safe by the US Food and Drug Administration (FDA) and the European Food Safety Authority (EFSA). However, LAB may act as intrinsic or extrinsic reservoirs for antibiotic resistance (AR) genes. This fact may not constitute a safety concern itself, as the resistance gene transfer is vertical. Nevertheless, external genetic elements may induce changes that favor the horizontal transfer transmission of resistance from pathogens as well as from the human intestinal microbiota, which represents a severe safety issue. Some genus of AR LAB includes *Enterococcus, Lactobacillus, Lactococcus, Leuconostoc, Pediococcus,* and *Streptococcus* isolated from fermented meat and milk products. Currently, the WHO recommends that LAB used in the food industry should be free of resistance. Therefore, the objective of this chapter is to present an overview of the LAB antibiotic resistance and some methods to determine the same.

**Keywords:** lactic acid bacteria, antibiotic resistance transfer, extrinsic genes, QPS strains, and GRAS

## 1. Introduction

The antimicrobial resistance has become one of the main safety issues for humanity, and several organizations, such as the World Health Organization (WHO), the Food and Agriculture Organization (FAO), the US Food and Drug Administration (FDA), and the European Food Safety Authority (EFSA) among others, have raised an awareness on this issue. The antimicrobial resistance can take place when microorganisms (bacteria, fungi, viruses, and parasites) are continuously exposed to antimicrobials (antibiotics, antivirals, antifungals, etc.), and as a result of an adaptation process, some microorganisms can survive and grow in the presence of the antimicrobial, which in normal conditions would inactivate them [1, 2]. In particular, antibiotics are drugs used to treat bacterial infections in humans and animals, preventing the reproduction of bacteria or inactivating them through several mechanisms (**Table 1**), either inhibiting the synthesis of the cell wall or the cytoplasmic membrane, blocking the protein synthesis or the DNA copying processes, altering the metabolism, or acting directly against the bacterial resistance pathway [3–5]. The use of antibiotics in humans (cephalosporins, broad-spectrum penicillins, and fluoroquinolones) has increased 36% from the years 2000 to 2010, mainly due to their inappropriate prescription and consumption for the treatment of viral instead of bacterial infections [3, 6]. This fact may be correlated with the global report on antimicrobial resistance that points over 700,000 human deaths each year associated to antimicrobial resistance, with a raising scenery to 10 million deaths each year by 2050 [2, 7].

The antimicrobial resistance involves several mechanisms associated to the presence of resistant genes that allow the direct inactivation of the active antimicrobial molecule as well as the loss of susceptibility to the antimicrobial by modification of the target site or reduction of the antimicrobial uptake [6]. Therefore, antimicrobials become ineffective, and resistant microorganisms can survive and transfer their resistant machinery to other microorganisms and

| *Site of action* | *Mode of action* | *Antibiotics* |
|---|---|---|
| Cell wall | Inhibition of precursors for the peptidoglycan synthesis | Fosfomycin<br>Cyloserine |
| | Stopping the transport of cell wall precursors through the membrane cell | Bacitracin<br>Mueridomycins |
| | Blocking the polymerization and crosslinking processes of wall peptidoglycan at the level of penicillin binding proteins (PBP's) | β-Lactams (penicillin derivates, cephalosporins, etc.), glycopeptides (vancomycin and teicoplanin) |
| Cytoplasmic membrane | Increasing the membrane permeability with the subsequent loss of small metabolites. | Polymyxins |
| | Depolarization of cytoplasmic membrane that reduces the protein and DNA synthesis | Lipopetides (daptomycin) |
| | Alteration of the membrane by formation of pores | Ionophores (valinomycin, tirocydins) and gramicydins |
| Protein synthesis | Inactivation of the protein activation process | Mupirocin, |
| | Inhibition of the protein synthesis initiation | Oxazolidiones and aminoglycosides |
| | Blocking the tRNA amino acid complex to ribosomes | Tetracycline and glycylcyclines |
| | Modification of the protein final elongation stages by blocking the peptidyl transferase on the 50S ribosome subunit | Amphenicols, lincosamides, macrolides, ketolides |
| DNA synthesis | Alteration of the DNA copying processes at the DNA-dependent RNA polymerase | Nitroimidazoles and nitrofurans |
| | Inactivation final DNA coiling process | Quinolones |
| Resistance mechanisms | Protects against bacterial enzyme β-lactamases that provide resistance to β-lactam antibiotics and/or blocks the antibiotic active efflux process. | Clavulanic acid, sulbactam and tazobactam |

**Table 1.** Antibiotics: Site and mode of action [3–5].

become a threat to public health [1]. The presence of antimicrobial-resistant microorganisms not only affects both the human and animal health but also increases the risk for spread and contamination of foods, crops, livestock, and aquaculture [3].

In particular, the FAO claims that 27 different antimicrobial classes are being frequently used in animals without an accurate reporting system to collect data related to their use and control [2]. Therefore, the WHO partners initiated a campaign all around the world in 2017, to raise the awareness of the antimicrobial resistance as part of a global program [1, 2]. The campaign constitutes a global action that involves governments, health professionals, food and feed industrialists, and the society to learn about antibiotic and antimicrobial resistance. It also includes some guidelines for the prevention and control of resistant *Enterobacteriaceae*, *Acinetobacter*, and *Pseudomonads* in health-care facilities. Additionally, the WHO recommends to farmers and the food industry sector to stop using antibiotics in healthy animals, in order to preserve the effectiveness of antibiotics currently used in human medicine [1–3, 8]. The global action plan on antimicrobial resistance points out that this issue has become an increasingly serious threat to public health and to the sustainable food production, where a rapid and effective response should involve the society and governments, as well as the health, food, and agriculture sectors and environmental specialists to promote practices that avoid the spread of antimicrobial resistance among common pathogens, especially those responsible for nosocomial and common infections [1, 2, 8].

The growing world population results in an increased demand for food, where antimicrobials such as antibiotics and fungicides are frequently used to treat infections in food-producing animals (cattle, swine, poultry, and fish), as well as in crops, to prevent diseases and as growth promoters [3]. This practice is frequently seen in developing countries where unauthorized high amounts of antibiotics are used that have been associated to the occurrence of multiple antibiotic-resistant *Enterococcus* and *Lactobacillus* strains from Indian poultry [2, 3, 9]. The FAO also reports that 90% of antibiotics may be excreted into the water and soil thus contaminating the environment, with the consequent exposure increment and development of AR microorganisms that can transfer their resistant genes to other microorganisms [2]. For instance, bacterial populations from the intestine of animals exposed to antibiotics (tetracycline, penicillin, sulfonamide, and polymyxins) were five times more likely to be resistant [6]. The resistant microorganisms can be spread to humans from contaminated foods and water or from the environment [2, 3]. Various practices such as adequate animal vaccination and the use of additives that promote health and efficiency of feed conversion, in combination with good hygiene and husbandry practices would reduce the need for antimicrobials and antibiotics for food production [7, 8].

Lactic acid bacteria (LAB) constitute one of the most important groups of microorganisms present in several habitats; they are in large numbers in the gastrointestinal tract of animals and humans and form part of the microbiota in several foods. Historically, LAB have been recognized as safe with a GRAS (generally recognized as safe) and QPS (qualified presumption of safety) status given by the FDA and EFSA authorities. However, the recent detection of antibiotic-resistant LAB and the continuous exposure to environmental conditions may promote that LAB became as intrinsic or extrinsic reservoirs for AR genes, which can be horizontally transmissible to pathogens through the food chain [3, 6]. The resistance to a specific antimicrobial may be intrinsic (when a microorganism does not possess target sites for the antimicrobial) or acquired. The acquired resistance is more complex and involves the presence of enzymes that inactivate the antimicrobial, posttranscriptional, or posttranslational modifications of the target site or reduction uptake and active efflux of the antimicrobial; those mechanisms derive from the gain of exogenous DNA or the mutation of indigenous DNA [4, 9, 10]. In general the AR genes can be horizontally transferred from one microorganism to another by transduction (via bacteriophages) or by transformation between microorganisms (when released DNA is taken up by other microorganism). However, it is claimed that the primary mechanism to acquire resistant is by direct cell to cell contact or conjugation between different genera of bacteria, especially when the resistant genes are present on mobile genetic elements such as plasmids and transposons [5, 10, 11]. LAB are highly adaptable and capable of developing resistance to antibiotics; most AR studies were focused on pathogenic microorganisms, but recently some investigators have questioned the safety of commensal LAB as some strains of *Lactococcus lactis*, *Enterococci*, and *Lactobacillus* isolated from fermented foods showed genes conferring resistance to tetracycline, erythromycin, and vancomycin [12].

Bacterial resistance to antibiotics is an emerging public concern that may compromise the efficacy of agents used for the treatment of infectious diseases [13]. Therefore, the objective of this chapter is to present an overview of the LAB antibiotic resistance and some methods to determine this characteristic, as per the FAO/OMS guideline for testing food-related bacteria and probiotics for resistance patterns.

## 2. Lactic acid bacteria

The term lactic acid bacteria refers to a taxonomically diverse group of Gram-positive bacteria, facultative anaerobic, nonspore-forming, nonmotile, and acid-tolerant cocci, coccobacilli, or rods that appear as single cells or forming couples, tetrads, or long chains, with common metabolism and physiology capable of fermenting sugars primarily into lactic acid. LAB species are found in two phyla, the *Firmicutes* and the *Actinobacteria*; for the first the genus, *Aerococcus*, *Alloiococcus*, *Carnobacterium*, *Enterococcus*, *Lactobacillus*, *Leuconostoc*, *Oenococcus*, *Pediococcus*, *Streptococcus*, *Tetragenococcus*, *Vagococcus*, and *Weissella* that are low G + C (31–49%) belong to the *Bacilli class* and the *Lactobacillales* order. While, the *Bifidobacterium* genus with a high G + C content (58–61%) belongs to the *Actinobacteria* phylum [6, 14, 15].

This bacterial group is classified into homofermentative and heterofermentative according to the end products derived from the glucose metabolism. The homofermentative converts glucose mainly into lactic acid by the Embden-Meyerhof pathway, while the heterofermentative LAB transforms glucose into lactic acid, carbon dioxide, and ethanol or acetic acid by the 6-phosphogluconate pathway. LAB are capable of inhibiting the growth of spoilage and pathogenic bacteria based on the competition for nutrients and adhesion niches due to their great acid tolerance and ability to adapt to redox changes [14, 15]. In addition LAB are capable to produce antimicrobial metabolites such as lactic and acetic acids, ethanol, hydrogen peroxide, diacetyl, antifungals (short-chain fatty acids derived from lipolysis reactions), antimicrobial peptides known as bacteriocins, and other antibacterial proteins like peptidoglycan hydrolases (PGH) capable to cleave the peptidoglycan cell wall of Gram-positive and Gram-negative bacteria [6, 14]. Bacteriocins are ribosomal antimicrobial peptides active against closely related and non-related sensitive bacterial strains by forming pores in the cytoplasmic membrane and responsible for the reduction of microbial LAB competitors under stress conditions. Several studies have demonstrated the potential of bacteriocins to be applied for food preservation and in the pharmaceutical industry for their action against spoilage microorganisms and pathogens such *Listeria monocytogenes* and *Staphylococcus aureus* [16–18].

LAB have been safely used for centuries in numerous indigenous food fermentations up to the actual modern industry in the elaboration processes for dairy products, vegetables, meats, coffee, cocoa, silages, sourdough bread, and wine, as LAB contribute to the taste, flavor, and texture of those fermented products but also inhibit the development of spoilage and pathogenic microorganism by acidification and production of antimicrobials [14, 19]. Therefore, LAB are widely employed as starter cultures in the food industry to accelerate ripening or to control the adventitious microbiota for elaboration and preservation of several fermented foods including dairy (hard- and semihard-type cheeses, yogurt, butter, and cream), meats, sourdough bread, and vegetables. LAB contribute to the taste, flavor, and texture of those fermented products as a result of several reactions, including lipolysis, proteolysis, and conversion of lactose in citrate and pyruvate intermediates that can be converted to various aromatic compounds, such as diacetyl, acetoin, acetaldehyde, and acetic acid. Proteolytic processes induces the accumulation of small peptides and free amino acids that are further transformed into alcohols, aldehydes, acids, and esters responsible for the flavor profile and organoleptic characteristics of fermented foods [14]. In addition some LAB strains such as *Lactococcus lactis, Lactobacillus sakei, Lactobacillus rhamnosus, Lactobacillus helveticus*, and *Streptococcus thermophilus* can produce exopolysaccharides (EPS) that not only confer protection to the cell producer but can be applied in the food industry as thickeners to increase viscosity and firmness, improving texture and mouthfeel of yogurt and other low-fat milk products. The EPS produced by LAB range from 10 to >2000 kDa and can be classified as homo- or heteropolysaccharides according to their monomer composition, where galactose, glucose, and rhamnose are the most common monomers [20].

Some LAB are present in the respiratory, gastrointestinal, and genital tracts of humans and animals and therefore used as probiotics for healthiness improvement related to their influence on the immune system for the prevention and control of some infections during pregnancy or as part of the treatment for antibiotic-derived diarrhea, constipation, and intestinal inflammation, also to manage allergies and lactose intolerance and prevention of urinary infections [21–23]. The WHO and FAO describe the probiotics as live microorganisms that in adequate amounts confer health benefits for the host [24]. Several strains of *Lactoccocus, Lactobacillus, Streptococcus, Enterococcus, Bifidobacterium, Pediococcus*, and *Propionibacteria* present in foods and in dietary supplements are commonly used as probiotics and considered desirable members of the intestinal microbiota that can be used to deliver vaccines and other metabolites directly in the gastrointestinal tract [21]. Consumption of LAB probiotics may help for modulation of the immune system and reduction of pathogens, thereby, improving the gut functionality. Other health benefits associated to the consumption of LAB probiotics include an antihypertensive effect, reduction in the serum cholesterol level, antioxidant effect, protection against colon cancer, reduction in the allergy symptoms, reduction in dental caries, and reduction in the obesity index [21, 22]. In addition, secondary metabolites with health-promoting properties include the antihypertensive angiotensin-converting enzyme produced through the proteolytic system of *Lactobacillus helveticus*, *Lactobacillus acidophilus*, and *Lactobacillus delbrueckii* [14, 22].

LAB are considered naturally resistant to several antibiotics and may have the potential to acquire resistance to other antimicrobials or to disseminate the resistance to pathogens present in the gastrointestinal tract of animals and humans [9]. For instance, Shao et al. [11] demonstrated that two isolates of *L. plantarum* possessed the *aaad*A and *ant*(6) genes associated to the resistance to streptomycin, and the overexposure to this antibiotic dramatically increased the minimum inhibitory concentration (MIC) and increased a cross-resistance to other antibiotics from the same class. On the other hand, the presence of 6% strains isolated from some pharmaceutical and dairy products from Egypt with tetracycline [*tet*(M)] and/or erythromycin [*erm*(B)] resistant genes has been reported [21]. In a similar study, a high incidence of *Lactobacillus* resistant to vancomycin (58%), erythromycin (10.8%), tetracycline (4.3%), gentamicin (48%), and ciprofloxacin (26%) was reported in Turkish fermented dairy products [13]. However, studies made by Flores and Mayo [25] indicate that no transfer of the tetracycline [*tet*(M)] and erythromycin [*erm*(B)] resistant genes from *S. thermophilus* to *L. delbrueckii* was detected during the production and storage of yogurt. Furthermore, the food chain can facilitate the transmission of antibiotic-resistant bacteria between animals, foods, and humans, being the fermented milk and meat products the most common vehicle for antibiotic-resistant bacteria to the indigenous flora of the gastrointestinal tract, as these products are consumed without a thermal treatment [12]. Even though that some reports confirm the transmission of resistant determinants, the two most common resistant genes in LAB are tetracycline [*tet*(M)] and erithromycin [*erm*(B)] resistant genes, followed by *cat* genes coding for chloramphenicol resistance [26]. Considering the wide range of potential applications of LAB in the industry and in the human and animal health, there is a need of their detailed examination that involves the detection of AR genes.

## 3. Transfer mechanisms of antibiotic resistance genes

For antibiotics to function and inhibit microbial growth, they must be at the proper concentration so that they can cross the cellular wall and interact with their target. As previously mentioned, AR is the capacity that has a microorganism to resist the inhibitory activity of an antibiotic beyond the normal susceptibility of similar bacterial species [27]. On the other hand, the different mechanisms of AR are based on the modification of the antibiotic target site as well as on the reduction of the antibiotic concentration that manages to get the cell target.

LAB are considered carriers of resistance genes that could propagate their genes within the food chain between food and humans, as well as to the environment through different mechanisms [27–30]. According to the FAO and WHO [24], it is important to determine whether starter or probiotic cultures intended for human or animal consumption have mobile resistance genes that could be transferred to other microorganisms [6, 31]. In addition, some authors have demonstrated that the use of antibiotics in animals destined for consumption, either as growth

http://dx.doi.org/10.5772/intechopen.80624

promoters or pathogen inhibitors, is directly related to the presence of AR microbiota in the human gastrointestinal tract [27, 32]. On the other hand, Gad et al. [21] isolated some *Lactobacillus, Streptococcus,* and *Lactococcus* strains from both pharmaceutical and probiotic dairy products, but the AR tests from the pharmaceutical probiotic isolates were free of resistance genes, unlike the LAB isolated from dairy products that showed resistance profiles comparable to those from pathogens such as *Staphylococcus spp., Escherichia coli,* and *Salmonella spp.* Furthermore, some *Enterococcus faecium* strains have demonstrated the transference of vancomycin resistant genes from to *Lactobacillus acidophilus* La5 "in vitro" and "in vivo" studies in the gut mice [33].

Exposure to antibiotics may allow bacteria to develop different mechanisms to counteract the bactericidal effect; a single bacterium can develop different types of resistance; these systems include an intrinsic or innate and the acquired resistance mode. Among these, the mechanism that prevails within bacteria varies according to the nature of the antibiotic, the target site, the bacterial species, and/or whether the resistance gene is part of the chromosome or mobile elements such as plasmids or transposons [12, 19, 28].

### 3.1. Mechanisms of resistance in LAB

Two relevant elements must be present for the antibiotic-target interaction, first the antibiotic must recognize the target, and the concentration of the antibiotic in the target must be sufficient to inhibit the bacterial growth. A resistance mechanism conduces to the antibiotic failure to inhibit the bacterial growth due to an inefficient antibiotic-target interaction, which can be classified as passive and active. The passive mechanism can only be transferred to other cells by clonal transfer that involves modifications of the target site or decrease in antimicrobial absorption, without affecting the antibiotic structure; this resistance is also known as intrinsic resistance. In contrast, the active mechanism involves the reduction on the concentration of the intracellular antibiotic by modification or degradation of its structure with enzymes or through the action of efflux pumps [34, 35].

**Figure 1** shows the mechanisms by which some bacteria can show resistance to antibiotics that involves (1) modification of the antibiotic by enzymatic complexes that prevent the antibiotic-target interaction, (2) enzymatic degradation of intra- or extracellular antibiotics, and (3) reduction in the intracellular antibiotic concentration through the activation of flow pumps or due to the change in the cell wall permeability [19].

The main mechanism of resistance to antibiotics presented by LAB has been related with multidrug-resistant (MDR) efflux pumps involved in the expulsion of structurally unrelated compounds [31, 36]. Wacher-Rodarte et al. [37] analyzed LAB isolated from pozol (a traditional fermented maize beverage), identifying that MDR strains such as *Lactococcus lactis* and *Lactobacillus plantarum* present active efflux pumps, including the chromosomally encoded ABC type with the LmrA transporter (*lmrA* gene). On the other hand, Poelarends et al. [38] demonstrated that the presence of the LmrA transporter in *Lactococcus lactis* is associated with the innate resistance of 17 up to 21 clinically relevant antibiotics, including aminoglycosides (kanamycin and gentamicin), lincosamines (clindamycin), macrolides (erythromycin), quinolones (ciprofloxacin), and tetracyclines. Other authors such as Casado Muñoz et al. [39] reported that *Lactobacillus pentosus* and *Leuconostoc pseudomesenteroides* isolated from fermented olives are resistant to cephalosporins, streptomycin, and kanamycin due to the

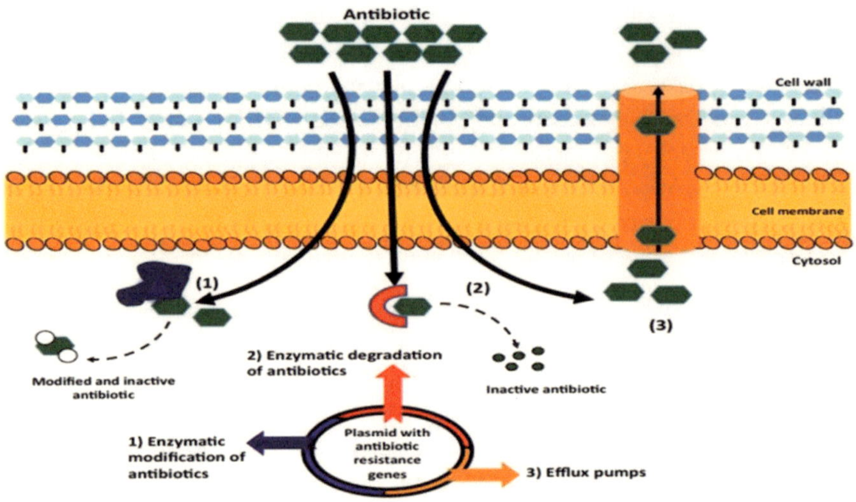


**Figure 1.** Mechanisms of antibiotic resistance in the LAB: (1) enzymatic modification, (2) enzymatic degradation, and (3) enzyme efflux pumps. Adapted from Sharma et al. [19].

variation of the cell wall permeability as their main mechanism of resistance; they also pointed that both strains presented a complex AcrAB-TolC system involved in MDR efflux pumps for β-lactams, fluoroquinolones, chloramphenicol, tetracycline, and other genes related with chromosomally encoded superfamily pumps *norA* and *Mde* that confer resistance to chloramphenicol and fluoroquinolones.

The resistance to aminoglycosides in LAB has not been reported, although in recent years LAB isolated from farm origin show resistant to gentamicin, kanamycin, and streptomycin, whose resistance mechanism is associated to impaired transport or enzymatic inactivation by three main aminoglycoside-modifying enzymes (AMEs) as N-acetyltransferases (AACs), O-phosphotransferases (APHs), and O-nucleotidyltransferases (ANTs) encoded by MGEs (mobile genetic elements) like transposons and insertion sequences [40].

Some bacteria belonging to the genera *Enterococcus*, *Lactobacillus*, *Pediococcus*, and *Bifidobacterium* present both intrinsic or innate and extrinsic or acquired AR, which can be a factor of food safety as they can spread resistance to other bacteria by vertical (between species) or horizontal transference (between bacterial genera) [25, 29, 31, 41].

#### *3.1.1. Intrinsic resistance*

Intrinsic resistance is the natural or innate ability of a bacterium to survive the effect of antibiotics, as a result of mutations derived from changes in the bacterial physiological state or by the uncontrolled exposure to antibiotics [42]. Intrinsic resistance has a minimum propagation potential between bacterial genera, as resistance genes are located into the chromosome with a limited transference to other genus, which represents a low risk within nonpathogenic bacteria. Any gene responsible for intrinsic resistance could be disseminated and transferred to other bacteria if it is flanked by insertion sequences that may promote its mobilization [12]. For instance, *Bifidobacterium* strains are commonly used as starter cultures and/or prebiotics in traditional and industrialized fermented foods although they have intrinsic resistance to quinolones (ciprofloxacin and nalidixic acid), mupirocin, tetracyclines, and aminoglycosides such as streptomycin; however, all the genes are located in the chromosome with a limited transference to other genus [28, 43]. It has been reported that some LAB genera have intrinsic resistance to bacitracin, vancomycin, kanamycin, teicoplanin, and quinolones [28]. This intrinsic resistance mechanisms presented by LAB include:

- Modification of the cell wall, commonly observed in the resistance to glycopeptides (vancomycin and teicoplanin) and non-ribosomal antibiotics (bacitracin). In particular, *Lactobacillus plantarum* and *Enterococcus faecium* present innate resistance to vancomycin, due to the substitution of D-alanine residues of the muramyl pentapeptide cell wall by D-lactate (high-level resistance) or D-serine (low-level resistance) in the chemical structure of the peptidoglycan, thus avoiding the antibiotic interaction [35, 41, 44].
- Enzymatic inactivation such as for aminoglycosides (neomycin, kanamycin, streptomycin) or quinolones (ciprofloxacin, norfloxacin, nalidixic acid) prevents the binding of these antibiotics with their specific targets, as observed for *Lactobacillus* and *Enterococcus* for the 16S rRNA of the 30S ribosomal bacterial subunit and DNA gyrase, respectively, that explains the intrinsic resistance to both groups of antibiotics [29, 40].

#### 3.1.2. *Extrinsic resistance*

Extrinsic or acquired resistance is one in which bacteria can incorporate into their cellular structure mobile genetic material capable of conferring resistance to certain antibiotics. Unlike intrinsic resistance, the acquired resistance is only found in some traits or bacterial subpopulations. The gene propagation may occur between bacteria of different genera or between different organisms. The horizontal gene transfer (HGT) occurs when the bacteria is capable of acquiring new genes that can increase their intrinsic resistance spectrum, or they can transfer resistance to other microorganisms or directly to humans or animals, which is already considered a health risk, according to the WHO. Therefore, the protocols for the analysis of resistance genes in LAB are increasing as they have a high capacity to acquire AR and since they have a close relationship with food processing [6, 19, 31, 45, 46]. **Figure 2** shows the three main mechanisms of HGT; some of which are not considered relevant in the transfer of resistance to antibiotics in LAB, for example, transduction (through bacteriophages) and transformation (when DNA is released from one bacterium and is absorbed by another), as the conjugation is the primary mechanism observed in lactic acid bacteria [12, 19, 47, 48].

The conjugation is the transfer of mobile genetic material from plasmids or transposons through a tube of proteins, called sexual pilus [6]. Plasmids are extrachromosomal DNA molecules capable of autonomous replication and that may confer resistance to microorganisms against antibiotics and represent one of the main mobile elements for dissemination of antibiotic-resistant genes against β-lactams, aminoglycosides, tetracyclines, chloramphenicol, sulfonamides, trimethoprim, macrolides, and quinolones [29, 47, 48].

Plasmids have a large number of genetic determinants that may confer resistance by conjugation, and it is important to consider that a single bacterium can have multiple plasmids [49].

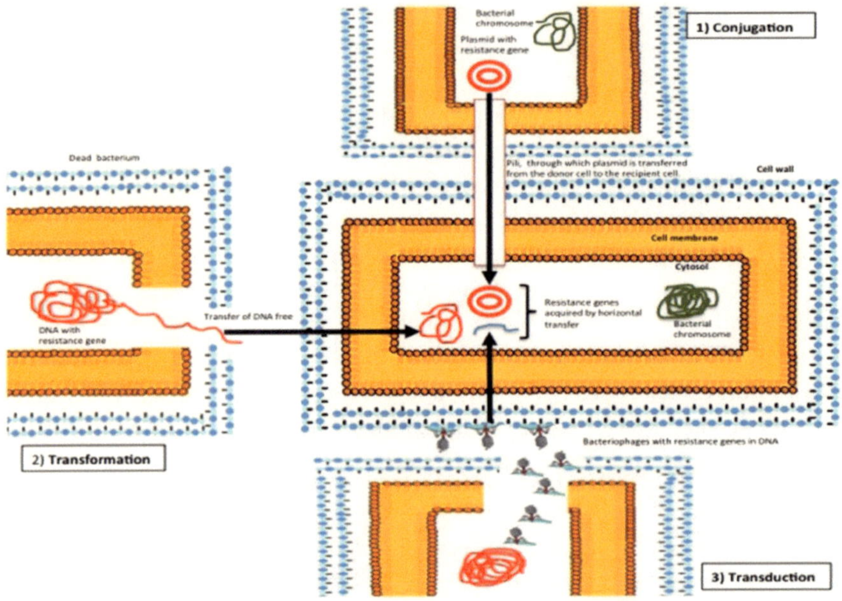


**Figure 2.** Mechanisms of horizontal gene transfer in the LAB. (1) conjugation is a process requiring the cell to cell contact via cell surface pili; (2) cell transformation by integrating extracellular DNA; (3) transduction, bacteriophages may transfer bacterial DNA from a previously infected donor cell to the recipient cell. Adapted from Sharma et al. [19] and Von Wintersdorff et al. [47].

Some authors indicate that the genetic diversity of resistance is proportional to the number of plasmids present in the environment, without forgetting that there are other mobile elements such as transposons and integrons, although these elements do not self-replicate and must be transported by an appropriate plasmid or phage [49, 50]. Some conjugative transposons used as vehicle of antibiotic resistance genes in LAB include Tn*916*, Tn*918*, Tn*920*, Tn*925*, Tn*2702* *(E. faecalis*), Tn*5233* (*E. faecium*), Tn*5276*, and Tn*5301* *(Lactococcus lactis*) [19].

### 3.2. Resistance to antibiotics in LAB

As mentioned, the presence of resistance genes in LAB is considered a public health problem, so the EFSA through the panel of additives and products or substances used in animal feed (FEEDAP) developed a technical guide to identify the bacteria that show acquired resistance to antibiotics such as ampicillin, vancomycin, gentamicin, kanamycin, streptomycin, erythromycin, clindamycin, tetracyclines, and chloramphenicol [51]. Most LAB that present acquired resistance in the food production chain include the obligate homofermentative *Lactobacillus* genera (*L. helveticus, L. acidophilus, L. delbrueckii*), obligate heterofermentative *Lactobacillus* (*L. reuteri, L. fermentum*), heterofermentative *Lactobacillus* facultative (*L. plantarum, L. rhamnosus, L. paracasei*), *Lactococcus lactis, Streptococcus thermophilus, Pediococcus spp., Leuconostoc spp.*, and *Enterococcus spp*. [31, 51]. On the other hand, LAB can be incorporated into food in the form of probiotic or starter cultures or they can be part of the natural microbiota of traditional fermented foods, but some authors have found that the vast majority of these bacteria are resistant to antibiotics [6, 19, 31, 40, 45]. **Table 2** shows some AR LAB isolated from traditional fermented foods, industrialized and probiotic recommended for improving the intestinal microbiota [20, 37, 49, 50].

In particular, the enterococcal and *Lactobacillus* genera may be associated to a health risk, as they carry innate and acquired resistance genes and because of their high residence in food and in the gastrointestinal microbiome of humans and animals [28, 36].

### 3.2.1. Enterococcus

Enterococci are widely distributed in vegetables, dairy products, prepared foods, and meat products and used as probiotics; however, they have intrinsic resistance to a large number of antibiotics such as β-lactams and aminoglycosides. In some cases, they can present profiles of resistance similar to enterococci considered nosocomial emergent pathogens which could present multiple drug resistance (MDR) with mechanisms of resistance that include modification of pharmacological targets, inactivation of therapeutic agents, overexpression of efflux pumps, and sophisticated adaptive response of cell envelope that promotes survival in the human host [41, 52].

| Lactic acid bacteria | Antibiotic resistance* | Food |
|---|---|---|
| *Lactobacillus sakei*<br>*Laactobacillus curvatus*<br>*Leuconostoc mesenteroides* | Vancomycin, gentamicin, ampicillin erythromycin and tetracyclines. | Chorizo, fuet and sausage |
| *Lactobacillus sakei*<br>*Pediococcus pentosaceus*<br>*Lactobacillus plantarum*<br>*Lactobacillus paraplantarum* | Streptomycin, gentamicin and tetracyclines. | Italian sausage |
| *Lactobacillus sakei*<br>*Lactobacillus plantarum* | Chloramphenicol, quinupristin-dalfopristin, lincomycin, erythromycin (*ermA, ermB* and *ermC*), rifampicin, tetracycline (*tet M, tetO, tetS, tetW, tetK and tetL* genes), gentamicin, vancomycin and penicillin. | Traditional dry fermented sausages from the south Portugal |
| *Enterococcus faecium*<br>*Enterococcus faecalis*<br>*Lactobacillus reuteri*<br>*Lactobacillus acidophilus*<br>*Lactobacillus delbrueckii subsp. bulgaricus*<br>*Lactobacillus johnsonii*<br>*Lactobacillus plantarum* | Gentamicin, tetracycline (*tetM*), clindamycin, vancomycin (*vanA*), chloramphenicol (*cat gen*), ciprofloxacin, penicillin and nitrofurantoin. | Sausages |
| *Lactococcus lactis* K214 | Chloramphenicol, streptomycin and tetracycline (*tetS* and *tetM)*, erythromycin (*ermT*). | Raw milk cheese |
| *Streptococcus thermophilus* | Tetracyclines (*tetS*), erythromycin (*ermB*), clindamycin, streptomycin and neomycin. | Raw milk |
| *Lactobacillus pentosus*<br>*Leuconostoc pseudomesenteroides* | Amoxicillin, ampicillin, chloramphenicol, gentamicin, erythromycin, streptomycin, vancomycin and teicoplanin. | Green olives |
| *Bifidobacterium spp.*<br>*Lactobacillus spp.*<br>*Streptococcus thermophilus* | Vancomycin, streptomycin, aztreonamine, gentamicin, ciprofloxacin, gentamicin, and ciprofloxacin. | Commercial probiotics |

**Italic letters indicate the resistance genes identified by Polymerase Chain Reaction (PCR).*

**Table 2.** Lactic acid bacteria resistant to antibiotics isolated from food [20, 37, 49, 50].

Streptomycin was the first aminoglycoside reported for which resistance appeared in enterococcal strains (concentrations higher than 2000 μg/mL); this resistance is carried out by adenylation of streptomycin, by the action of the enzyme streptomycin adenyltransferase, encoded by the *aadA* gene [35, 41]. Resistance to gentamicin, kanamycin, neomycin, and netilmicin (aminoglycosides as well) is mainly due to the production of the bifunctional enzyme 2′-phosphotransferase-6′-acetyltransferase, which promotes the ATP-dependent phosphorylation of aminoglycosides [41].

Strains of enterococci of clinical origin between 60 and 65% exhibit resistance to tetracyclines, although these antibiotics are not routinely used in the treatment of infections caused by these microorganisms. There are two fundamental mechanisms of resistance to tetracyclines in enterococci: flow pumps and protection of the ribosome, thus preventing the binding of the antibiotic. The *tetK* and *tetL* genes code for proteins associated to flow pumps responsible to remove the antibiotic outside of the cell, while the *tetM, tetO,* and *tetS* genes code for proteins that provide resistance to tetracyclines for ribosome protection. The *tetL* and *tetM* genes are the most frequent in the chromosome and mobile determinants [41, 52, 53]. Finally, vancomycin (glycopeptide) is the main cause of concern, since this antibiotic is considered at the last option for antibiotic therapy for the treatment of Gram-positive bacteria. The resistance to vancomycin in enterococci is varied, having described six genotypes called *vanA, vanB, vanC, vanD, vanE,* and *vanG,* where the genotype *vanA* is more frequent in the *Enterococcus* genus [41].

#### 3.2.2. *Lactobacillus*

In general, Lactobacilli have a high natural resistance to vancomycin, bacitracin, cefoxitin, metronidazole, nitrofurantoin, and sulfadiazine, as well as antibiotics that inhibit the synthesis of proteins such as chloramphenicol, erythromycin, quinupristin/dalfopristin, lincomycin, clindamycin, and tetracyclines [45]. Guo et al. [54] observed 85% of incidence of vancomycin resistance in food isolated *Lactobacillus* strains, especially in *Lactobacillus plantarum* and *Lactobacillus casei,* with the lower frequency for *Lactobacillus helveticus,* but these resistances are not transferable, as genes are located in the chromosome [54]. In addition, genes that code for resistance to tetracycline and erythromycin have been detected in different *Lactobacillus* species isolated of probiotics and foods [12, 31, 55].

The genus *Lactobacillus* is an excellent receptor for exogenous genes by conjugation, as demonstrated by Abriouel et al. [45] for the conjugative pAMβ1 plasmid found in *Lactobacillus plantarum* that could be obtained from enterococci and streptococci. *Lactobacillus* are commonly susceptible to antibiotics, such as penicillins (ampicillin, oxacillin, and piperacillin), inhibitors of β-lactamase, and cephalosporins (cephalothin and cefuroxime, ceftriaxone and cefoxitin), but in recent years some authors have reported resistance to penicillin G in some strains of *Lactobacillus rhamnosus, Lactobacillus reuteri,* and *Lactobacillus plantarum* [45, 56]. Other studies demonstrated that *Lactobacillus rhamnosus* is safe to use as a starter or probiotic culture, despite having resistance genes to vancomycin, as these resistance is encoded into the chromosome [45, 48, 54].

### 3.3. Horizontal transfer of LAB to the intestinal microbiota

The horizontal gene transfer (HGT) involves the gene interchange between different bacteria through mobile DNA elements such as plasmids, conjugative transposons, integrons, and bacteriophages [27, 47–49]. The transfer of resistance genes by HGT initiates from the farm animals that were treated with antibiotics used as growth promoters to prevent diseases, but these uncontrolled treatments may induce resistance in their intestinal microbiota; later this biota can reach foods and finally being transferred to the human [3]. Conjugation in food matrices has been reported from commensal bacterium (*Enterococcus faecalis* and *Lactococcus lactis*) to potentially pathogenic strains (*Listeria spp., Salmonella spp., Staphylococcus aureus*, and *E. coli*) in fermented milk [25, 27]. Also, the transfer of tetracycline resistance genes among LAB has been reported in fermented milk and fermented sausages [27]. Martínez and Baquero [34] report the HGT of tetracycline and vancomycin resistance genes in *Enterococcus faecalis* during the fermentation process of cheese and sausages. Bonham et al. [30] have demonstrated that aged cheeses contain AR *Lactobacillus* and *Lactococcus* that acquired the resistance through HGT induced by the strong condition of microbial selection during the food production and maturation process.

A wide diversity of AR species can be found in the human gastrointestinal tract that could be acquired AR genes by HGT; this fact is related to the metagenomic comparison showing that most resistance genes found in the human microbiome are those associated with approved antibiotics used in livestock, which supported the hypothesis that resistance genes can be transferred from the farm to consumers [48]. Therefore, the WHO indicates that the HGT genes can be a significant health problem, as most antibiotic resistance is acquired through the HGT [1].

## 4. Regulation of the use of LAB

The FDA categorizes microorganisms with the GRAS distinction after being evaluated in general aspects of safety, taxonomy, potential to produce pathogenicity toxins, resistance to antibiotics, and the historical background of food safety. LAB have a broad history of use in fermented foods and usually recognized as safe. However, the dissemination of AR genes puts the GRAS category in another context, especially for bacteria that present mobile genes of transfer such as *Lactobacillus*, since in the US there are still no guidelines that contemplate the type of resistance in microorganism used in food processing [57]. On the other hand, the EU commission regulates the safety of LAB used as starter or probiotic cultures in the European continent, through the EFSA that establishes guidelines for assigning qualified presumption of safety quality to the organisms since 2003. As previously mentioned, the term QPS is based on reasonable and qualified evidence to allow certain restrictions and may be analogous to the GRAS concept but with more rigid guidelines in which the reliable safety of the bacteria is verified, making clear the phrase "from farm to fork" [58]. The QPS status is given to a bacterium, by the EFSA BIOHAZ Panel (Biological Hazards) that must take into account the following aspects (**Figure 3**): (1) the identity of the taxonomic unit at the genus level; (2) documentation related to the LAB safety, based on scientific evidence and history of use; (3) pathogenicity, in which it is evaluated if any species of the genus has pathogenicity factors, if the information is available, the pathogenic strains are excluded; and (4) knowledge of the final use of the microorganism, identifying if the bacteria is part of the food chain or if it is used to produce other products [6, 58].

The list of QPS includes species of *Lactobacillus sakei, Lactobacillus curvatus, Lactobacillus plantarum, Lactobacillus fermentum, Lactobacillus brevis, Lactobacillus rhamnosus, Lactobacillus*

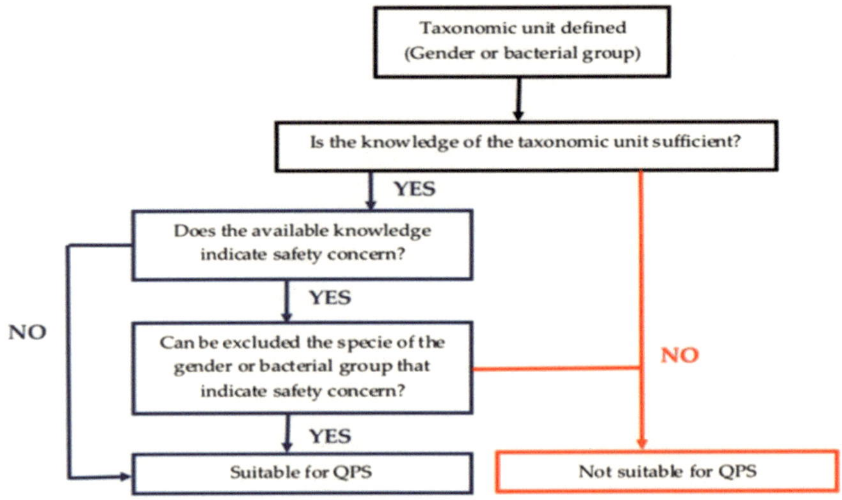


**Figure 3.** Scheme for assessing the suitability for qualified presumption of safety (QPS) status of a BAL. adapted from Laulund et al. [58].

*alimentarius, Leuconostoc lactis, Leuconostoc citreum, Leuconostoc mesenteroides, Leuconostoc pseudomesenteroides, Pediococcus acidilactici, Pediococcus dextrinicus, Pediococcus pentosaceus, Lactococcus lactis*, and *Streptococcus thermophilus* [6]. In the case of *Enterococcus*, the QPS category cannot be assigned to all species; each specie must be individually analyzed [6].

## 5. Methods to identify antibiotic-resistant LAB

Most widely used antibiotic susceptibility testing methods are based on (1) phenotypic detection of antibiotic resistance by measuring bacterial growth in the presence of the tested antibiotic and (2) molecular identification of resistant genotypes through polymerase chain reaction (PCR) [21, 25, 29, 39, 54]. The evaluation of phenotypic susceptibility to antibiotics in lactic acid bacteria should be done using recognized methods that allow the identification of the minimum inhibitory concentration (MIC) for the most commonly used antibiotics. Most LAB species used in food can be evaluated by the method described in ISO 10932: 2010 [59], considering the conditions and culture media for *Bifidobacteria* and LAB that do not belong to the genus enterococci [56, 57]. In case of having strains of *Enterococcus*, it is recommended to use the methods described by the Clinical and Laboratory Standards Institute [21, 60]. Some of the recommended methods to determine the MIC in LAB are the E-test, the Kirby-Bauer test (diffusion method), and the broth microdilution method (MDIL) [43]. In particular the cutoff values are known for the genera *Lactobacillus, Pediococcus, Lactococcus, Streptococcus*, and *Bifidobacteria*. The MDIL method is widely used to evaluate MIC for a large number of strains and antibiotics, although the method has some limitations, especially for those antibiotics for which a strain could quickly acquire resistance [43]. However, MIC evaluation in LAB is somewhat inconsistent among the researchers, mainly due to the lack of culture media that can ensure proper growth of LAB without interfering with the assay results. Therefore, a complementary technique involves the search for AR genes using PCR techniques and microarrays [25, 29, 54]. Also, identifying the location of these genes allows to determine their potential transfer, while their sequencing can provide evidence of their bacterial taxa and identity of the genes, which helps to trace the origin of their genomes [29].

Functional metagenomics is an important approach in the investigation of antibiotic resistance genes (ARG) since it can be used to identify and characterize new ARG, including those not previously associated with antibiotic resistance [48, 61]. It is also one of the most recent techniques in the study of resistance in pure bacterial groups or more complex samples such as food; some works reported in the literature indicate the wide diversity of resistance systems that are present in food, considering the cultivable and not cultivable bacteria. Metagenomic studies help to understand the mechanisms of resistance in such a way that it allows direct applications in the identification of new drugs and the synthesis of novel and active antibiotic molecules [61].

### 5.1. Procedure to evaluate LAB resistant to antibiotic used in food

The FEEDAP Panel proposed a scheme to evaluate the resistance present in lactic acid bacteria that can be used as probiotic or starter cultures in food processing; as previously mentioned, it is essential to distinguish between the intrinsic and acquired resistance as part of the food safety of lactic acid bacteria [58, 62]. The correct identification of the bacteria (sequencing and comparison of the 16S rDNA gene in international databases) by molecular taxonomy is essential to evaluate the type of resistance, since the intrinsic resistance is specific for a specie or genus. Once the specie under study has been identified, the MIC (minimum inhibitory concentration)

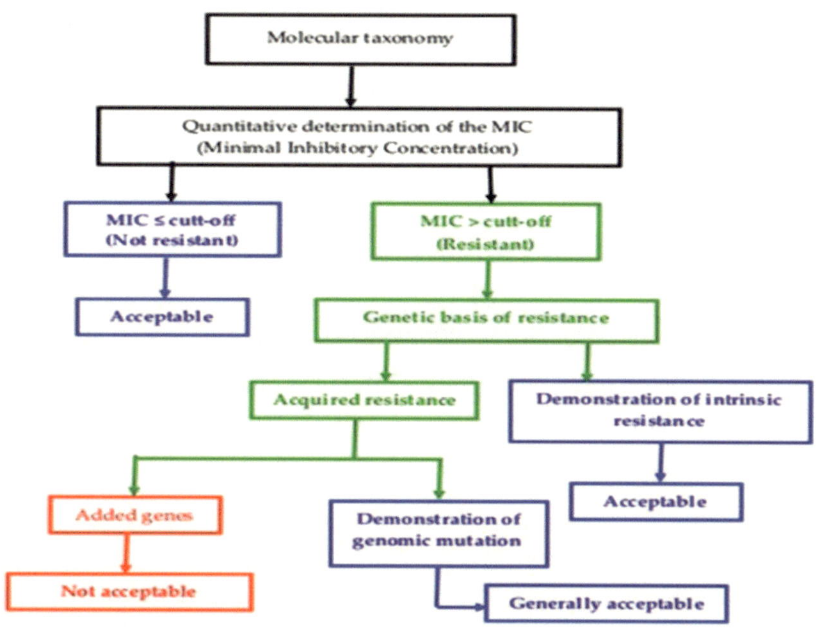


**Figure 4.** Proposed scheme for the antibiotic resistance assessment of lactic acid bacteria used as probiotic and starter culture. Adapted from Laulund et al. [58] and EFSA [62].

in which the LAB is sensitive to the antibiotic analyzed is determined. The bacterium can be considered safe when the MIC is lower than the cutoff level (MIC < cutoff). On the other hand, if the MIC value is above the cutoff value (MIC > cutoff), the bacterium is considered resistant to the antibiotic, and its resistance should be confirmed by molecular methods as PCR [39, 54, 62]. However, the resistance genes not always are expressed but can be transferred to other bacteria if the environmental conditions stimulate the expression of these genes [34]. If the bacteria have intrinsic resistance, it is considered acceptable for use in food. Otherwise, it must be demonstrated whether the acquired resistance is in mobile genetic material or was acquired in the process of mutation in the bacterial chromosome (also acceptable for use in foods). Finally, the bacteria are not accepted by any regulatory body for its application in food if it is demonstrated that the resistance is exogenous and easily transferable (**Figure 4**).

## 6. Conclusion

LAB are of great importance in the food industry for the preparation of fermented foods, in addition to being widely used as probiotics to regulate the intestinal microbiota in animals and humans. However, it is important to carry out the appropriate tests to identify the presence of antibiotic resistance genes that can be transferred horizontally to other microorganisms, whether pathogenic or those present in the gastrointestinal microbiota, which can cause a health problem because of the continuous exposure to the environmental conditions that favor the resistance spread that threats the public health and the food production.

## Conflict of interest

"No conflict of interest declared."

## Author details

Yenizey M. Álvarez-Cisneros and Edith Ponce-Alquicira*

*Address all correspondence to: pae@xanum.uam.mx

Departamento de Biotecnología, Universidad Autónoma Metropolitana, Unidad Iztapalapa, Mexico City, Mexico

## References

[1] World Health Organization. Global Action Plan on Antimicrobial Resistance. 2015. Available from: http://www.who.int/antimicrobial-resistance/publications/global-action-plan/en/ [Accessed: Jun 26, 2018] ISBN: 9789241509763

[2] Antimicrobial Resistance in Food and Agriculture. FCC-EMPRES, information sheets. April 2017. Available from: http://www.fao.org/antimicrobial-resistance [Accessed: Jun 26, 2018]

[3] Mermelstein NH. Combating antibiotic resistance. Food Technology. 2018;**72**(3):62-65

[4] Calvo M, Martínez LM. Antimicrobial mechanisms of action. Enfermedades Infecciosas y Microbiología Clínica. 2009;**27**:44-52. DOI: 10.1016/j.eimc.2008.11.001

[5] Kapoor G, Saigal S, Elongavan A. Action and resistance mechanisms of antibiotics: A guide for clinicians. Journal of Anaesthesiology Clinical Pharmacology. 2017;**33**(3):300-305. DOI: 10.4103/joacp.JOACP_349_15

[6] Fraqueza MJ. Antibiotic resistance of lactic acid bacteria isolated from dry-fermented sausages. International Journal of Food Microbiology. 2015;**212**:76-88. DOI: 10.1016/j.ijfoodmicro.2015.04.035

[7] O'Neill J. Tackling drug-resistant infections globally: Final report and recommendations. In: The Review on Antimicrobial Resistance. 2016. pp. 10-12. Available from: https://amr-review.org/ [Accessed: Jul 21, 2018]

[8] The FAO Action Plan on Antimicrobial Resistance 2016-2020. Rome: Food and Agriculture Organization of the United Nations; 2016. ISBN: 978-92-5-109392-4

[9] Preethi C, Rao-Thumu SC, Halami PM. Occurrence and distribution of multiple antibiotic-resistant *Enterococcus* and *Lactobacillus spp*. from Indian poultry: In vivo transferability of their erythromycin, tetracycline and vancomycin resistance. Annales de Microbiologie. 2017;**67**:395-340. DOI: 10.1007/s13213-017-1270-6

[10] Dowling A, Dwyer JO, Adley CC. Antibiotics: Mode of action and mechanisms of resistence. In Méndez-Vilas A, editor. Antimicrobial Research: Novel Bioknowledge and Educational Programs. 1st ed. Badajoz, Spain: Formatex Research Centre; 2017. 536 p. ISBN (13): 978-84-947512-0-2

[11] Shao Y, Zhang W, Guo H, Pan L, Zhang H, Sun T. Comparative studies on antibiotic resistance in *Lactobacillus casei* and *Lactobacillus plantarum*. Food Control. 2015;**50**:250-258. DOI: 10.1016/j.foodcont.2014.09.003

[12] Mathur S, Singh R. Antibiotic resistance in food lactic acid bacteria—A review. International Journal of Food Microbiology. 2005;**105**:281-295. DOI: 10.1016/j.ijfoodmicro.2005.03.008

[13] Erginkaya Z, Turhan EU. Determination of antibiotic resistance of lactic acid bacteria isolated for traditional Turkish fermented dairy products. Iranian Journal of Veterinary Research. 2018;**19**:53-56

[14] Giraffa G. Overview of the ecology and biodiversity of the LAB. In: Hotzapfel WH, Wood BJB, editors. Lactic Acid Bacteria: Biodiversity and Taxonomy. 1st ed. London: John Wiley; 2014. 45 p. DOI: 10.1002/9781118655252

[15] Khalid K. An overview of lactic acid bacteria. International Journal of Bioscience. 2011; **1**:1-13. ISSN: 2220-6655

[16] Schneider R, Fernandez FJ, Aguilar MB, Guerrero-Legarreta I, Alpuche-Solis A, Ponce-Alquicira E. Partial characterization of a class IIa pediocin produced by *Pediococcus parvulus* 133 strain isolated from meat (Mexican chorizo). Food Control. 2006;**17**:909-915. DOI: 10.1016/j.foodcont.2005.06.010

[17] Álvarez-Cisneros YM, Fernandez FJ, Wacher-Rodarte C, Aguilar MB, Sáinz-Espuñes TDR, Ponce-Alquicira E. Biochemical characterization of a bacteriocin-like inhibitory substance produced by *Enterococcus faecium* MXVK29, isolated from Mexican traditional sausage. Journal of Science and Food Agriculture. 2010;**90**:2475-2481. DOI: 10.1002/jsfa.4109

[18] Yang S-C, Lin C-H, Sung CT, Fang J-Y. Antibacterial activities of bacteriocins: Application in foods and pharmaceuticals. Frontiers in Microbiology. 2014;**5**:241. DOI: 10.3389/fmicb.2014.00241

[19] Sharma P, Tomar SK, Goswami P, Sangwan V, Singh R. Antibiotic resistance among commercially available probiotics. Food Research International. 2014;**57**:176-195. DOI: 10.1016/j.foodres.2014.01.025

[20] Vaningelgem F, Zamfir M, Mozzi F, Adriany T, Vancanneyt M, Swings J, et al. Biodiversity of exopolysaccharides produced by *Streptococcus thermophilus* strains is reflected in their production and their molecular and functional characteristics. Applied and Environmental Microbiology. 2004;**70**:900-912. DOI: 10.1128/AEM.70.2.900-912.2004

[21] Gad GFM, Abdel-Hamid AM, Farag ZSH. Antibiotic resistance in lactic acid bacteria isolated from some pharmaceutical and dairy products. Brazilian Journal of Microbiology. 2014;**45**:25-33

[22] Dicks LMT, Botes M. Probiotic lactic acid bacteria in the gastro-intestinal tract: Health benefits, safety and mode of action. Beneficial Microbes. 2010;**1**:11-29. DOI: 10.3920/BM2009.0012

[23] Lim IS, Lee HS, Kim WY. The effect of lactic acid bacteria isolates on the urinary tract pathogens to infants in vitro. Journal of Korean Medical Science. 2009;**24**:S57-S62. DOI: 10.3346/jkms.2009.24.S1.S57

[24] Report of a Join FAO/WHO Working Group on Drafting Guidelines for the Evaluation of Probiotics in Food. In: Probiotics in Food – Health and Nutritional Properties and Guidelines for Evaluation. Ontario, Canada; 2002. Rome: FAO Food and Nutrition Paper 85. 2006. pp. 39-52. ISBN: 92-5-105513-0

[25] Flórez A, Mayo B. Antibiotic resistance-susceptibility profiles of *Streptococcus thermophilus* isolated from raw milk and genome analysis of the genetic basis of acquired resistances. Frontiers in Microbiology. 2017;**8**:2680. DOI: 10.3389/fmicb.2017.02608

[26] Moračanin SV, Djukić D, Zdolec N, Milijašević M, Mašković P. Antimicrobial resistance of lactic acid bacteria in fermented food. Journal of Hygienic Engineering and Design. 2017;**18**:25-35 UDC 663.18:579.864

[27] Verraes C, Van Boxstael S, Van Meervenne E, Van Coillie E, Butaye P, Catry B, et al. Antimicrobial resistance in the food chain: A review. International Journal of Environmental Research and Public Health. 2013;**10**:2643-2669. DOI: 10.3390/ijerph10072643

[28] Imperial IC, Ibana JA. Addressing the antibiotic resistance problem with probiotics: Reducing the risk of its double-edged sword effect. Frontiers in Microbiology. 2016;**7**: 1983. DOI: 10.3389/fmicb.2016.01983

[29] Clementi F, Aquilanti L. Recent investigations and updated criteria for the assessment of antibiotic resistance in food lactic acid bacteria. Anaerobe. 2011;**17**:394-398. DOI: 10.1016/j.anaerobe.2011.03.021

[30] Bonham KS, Wolfe BE, Dutton RJ. Extensive horizontal gene transfer in cheese-associated bacteria. eLife. 2017;**6**:e.22144. DOI: 10.7554/eLife.22144

[31] Gueimonde M, Sánchez B, de los Reyes-Gavilán CG, Margolles A. Antibiotic resistance in probiotic bacteria. Frontiers in Microbiology. 2013;**4**:202. DOI: 10.3389/fmicb.2013.00202

[32] Forslund K, Sunagawa S, Kultima JR, Mende DR, Arumugam M, Typas A, et al. Country-specific antibiotic use practices impact the human gut resistome. Genome Research. 2013; **23**:1163-1169. DOI: 10.1101/gr.155465.113

[33] Mater DD, Langella P, Corthier G, Flores MJ. A probiotic *Lactobacillus* strain can acquire vancomycin resistance during digestive transit in mice. Journal of Molecular Microbiology and Biotechnology. 2008;**14**:123-127. DOI: 10.1159/000106091

[34] Martínez JL, Baquero F. Emergence and spread of antibiotic resistance: Setting a parameter space. Upsala Journal of Medical Sciences. 2014;**119**:68-77. DOI: 10.3109/03009734.2014.901444

[35] Munita JM, Arias CA. Mechanisms of antibiotic resistance. Microbiology Spectrum. 2016;**4**(2):1-37. DOI: 10.1128/microbiolspec.VMBF-0016-2015

[36] Mazurkiewicz P, Sakamoto K, Poelarends GJ, Konings WN. Multidrug transporters in lactic acid bacteria. Mini Reviews in Medicinal Chemistry. 2005;**5**:173-181. DOI: 10.2174/1389557053402675

[37] Wacher-Rodarte MC, Trejo-Muñúzuri TP, Montiel-Aguirre JF, Drago-Serrano ME, Gutiérrez-Lucas RL, Castañeda-Sánchez JI, et al. Antibiotic resistance and multidrug-resistant efflux pumps expression in lactic acid bacteria isolated from pozol, a nonalcoholic Mayan maize fermented beverage. Food Science & Nutrition. 2016;**4**(3):423-430. DOI: 10.1002/fsn3.304

[38] Poelarends GJ, Mazurkiewicz P, Konings WN. Multidrug transporters and antibiotic resistance in *Lactococcus lactis*. Biochimica et Biophysica Acta. 2002;**10**:1555. DOI: 10.1016/S0005-2728(02)00246-3

[39] Casado Muñoz MC, Benomar N, Lerma LL, Gálvez A, Abriouel H. Antibiotic resistance of *Lactobacillus pentosus* and *Leuconostoc pseudomesenteroides* isolated from naturally-fermented Aloreña table olives throughout fermentation process. International Journal of Food Microbiology. 2014;**172**:110-118. DOI: 10.1016/j.ijfoodmicro.2013.11.025

[40] Jaimee G, Halami PM. Emerging resistance to aminoglycosides in lactic acid bacteria of food origin-an impending menace. Applied Microbiology and Biotechnology. 2016; **100**:1137-1151. DOI: 10.1007/s00253-015-7184-y

[41] Miller WR, Munita JM, Arias CA. Mechanisms of antibiotic resistance in enterococci. Expert Review of Anti-infective Therapy. 2014;**12**:1221-1236. DOI: 10.1586/14787210.2014.956092

[42] Zhang Y. Advances in the treatment of tuberculosis. Clinical Pharmacology & Therapeutics. 2007;**82**:595-600. DOI: 10.1038/sj.clpt.6100362

[43] Kushiro A, Chervaux C, Cools-Portier S, Perony A, Legrain-Raspaud S, Obis D, et al. Antimicrobial susceptibility testing of lactic acid bacteria and bifidobacteria by broth microdilution method and Etest. International Journal of Food Microbiology. 2009;**132**: 54-58. DOI: 10.1016/j.ijfoodmicro.2009.03.012

[44] Zhang S, Oh J-H, Alexander LM, Özçam M, van Pijkeren J-P. D-Alanyl-D-alanine ligase as a broad-host-range counterselection marker in vancomycin-resistant lactic acid bacteria. Journal of Bacteriology. 2018;**200**:e00607-e00617. DOI: 10.1128/JB.00607-17

[45] Abriouel H, Casado Muñoz MD, Lerma LL, Perez Montoro B, Bockelman W, Pichner R, et al. New insights in antibiotic resistance of *Lactobacillus* species from fermented foods. Food Research International. 2015;**78**:465-481. DOI: 10.1016/j.foodres.2015.09.016

[46] Zheng M, Zhang R, Tian X, Zhou X, Pan X, Wong A. Assessing the risk of probiotic dietary supplements in the context of antibiotic resistance. Frontiers in Microbiology. 2017;**8**:908. DOI: 10.3389/fmicb.2017.00908

[47] Von Wintersdorff CJ, Penders J, van Niekerk JM, Mills ND, Majumder S, van Alphen LB, et al. Dissemination of antimicrobial resistance in microbial ecosystems through horizontal gene transfer. Frontiers in Microbiology. 2016;**7**:173. DOI: 10.3389/fmicb.2016.00173

[48] Huddleston JR. Horizontal gene transfer in the human gastrointestinal tract: Potential spread of antibiotic resistance genes. Infection and Drug Resistance. 2014;**7**:167-186. DOI: 10.2147/IDR.S48820

[49] Brown-Jaque M, Calero-Cáceres W, Muniesa M. Transfer of antibiotic-resistance genes via phage-related mobile elements. Plasmid. 2015;**79**:1-7. DOI: 10.1016/j.plasmid.2015.01.001

[50] Ma L, Li B, Zhang T. Abundant rifampin resistance genes and significant correlations of antibiotic resistance genes and plasmids in various environments revealed by metagenomic analysis. Applied Microbiology and Biotechnology. 2014;**98**:5195-5204. DOI: 10.1007/s00253-014-5511-3

[51] European Food Safety Authority (EFSA). Technical guidance-update of the criteria used in the assessment of bacterial resistance to antibiotics of human or veterinary importance. EFSA Journal. 2008;**732**:1-15. DOI: 10.2903/j.efsa.2008.732

[52] Álvarez-Cisneros YM, Fernández FJ, Sainz-Espuñez T, Ponce-Alquicira E. Assessment of virulence factors, antibiotic resistance and amino-decarboxylase activity in *Enterococcus faecium* MXVK29 isolated from Mexican chorizo. Letters in Applied Microbiology. 2017;**64**: 171-176. DOI: 10.1111/lam.12699

[53] Enayati M, Sadeghi J, Nahaei MR, Aghazadeh M, Pourshafie MR, et al. Virulence and antimicrobial resistance of *Enterococcus faecium* isolated from water samples. Letters in Applied Microbiology. 2015;**61**:339-345. DOI: 10.1111/lam.12474

[54] Guo H, Pan L, Li L, Lu J, Kwok L, Menghe B, et al. Characterization of antibiotic resistance genes from *Lactobacillus* isolated from traditional dairy products. Journal of Food Science. 2017;**3**:724-730. DOI: 10.1111/1750-3841.13645

[55] Devirgiliis C, Zinno P, Perozzi G. Update on antibiotic resistance in foodborne *Lactobacillus* and *Lactococcus* species. Frontiers in Microbiology. 2013;**4**:301. DOI: 10.3389/fmicb.2013.00301

[56] Wang J, Guo H, Cao C, Zhao W, Kwok LY, Zhang H, et al. Characterization of the adaptive amoxicillin resistance of *Lactobacillus casei* Zhang by proteomic analysis. Frontiers in Microbiology. 2018;**9**:292. DOI: 10.3389/fmicb.2018.00292

[57] Mattia A, Merker R. Regulation of probiotic substances as ingredients in foods: Premarket approval or "generally recognized as safe" notification. Clinical Infectious Diseases. 2008; **46**(supplement_2):S115-S118. DOI: 10.1086/523329

[58] Laulund S, Wind A, Derkx PM, Zuliani V. Regulatory and safety requirements for food cultures. Microorganisms. 2017;**5**:E28. DOI: 10.3390/microorganisms5020028

[59] International Organization for Standardization. ISO10932:2010 Milk and Milk Products—Determination of the Minimal Inhibitory Concentration (MIC) of Antibiotics Applicable to Bifidobacteria and Non-enterococcal Lactic Acid Bacteria (LAB). Geneva, Switzerland: International Organization for Standardization; 2010

[60] Laboratory Standards Institute. CLSI Guidelines. Available from: https://clsi.org/standards/products/microbiology/documents/m100/ [Accessed: Jun 26, 2018]

[61] Dos Santos DFK, Istvan P, Quirino BF, Kruger RH. Functional metagenomics as a tool for identification of new antibiotic resistance genes from natural environments. Microbial Ecology. 2017;**73**:479-491. DOI: 10.1007/s00248-016-0866-x

[62] Technical guidance prepared by the panel on additives and products or substance used in animal feed (FEEDAP) on the update of the criteria used in the assessment of bacterial resistance to antibiotics of humans or veterinary importance. EFSA Journal. 2008;**732**:1e15. DOI: 10.2903/j.efsa.2008.732

Chapter 5

# Development of Antibiotic Resistance in Wastewater Treatment Plants

Fateme Barancheshme and Mariya Munir

Additional information is available at the end of the chapter

http://dx.doi.org/10.5772/intechopen.81538

**Abstract**

Antibiotic resistant bacteria and antibiotic resistance genes have been of the emerging contaminant threatening human health. The overuse of antibiotics, both in human patients and, importantly, in livestock, has led to an explosion of antibiotic-resistant bacteria, both in the U.S. and around the world. The prediction from the World Health Organization (WHO) is that, if nothing changes, the future will look a lot like the past—where people die from minor injuries that become infected. One of the goals should be a long-term sustainable balance with everything in our environment, including bacteria to promote human health. Different microbial techniques have been employed to study the occurrence and spread of antibiotic resistance in the environment, preventing us from returning to a pre-antibiotic era. Dissemination of antibiotic resistance genes to the environment is an important factor causing an increased prevalence of resistant pathogens. Their spread to multidrug-resistant pathogens is one of the most emerging clinical challenges.

**Keywords:** antibiotic resistant genes, antibiotic resistant bacteria, wastewater, wastewater treatment plant, microbial pathogens

## 1. Introduction

Antibiotics have been used broadly in the last decades for disease control as well as livestock breeding. The misuse and inappropriate disposal of antibiotics can develop antibiotic resistance bacteria (ARB) and multi-drug resistant bacteria which carry one or more antibiotic resistance genes (ARGs). In this century, ARB and ARGs are known as emerging pollutants that threaten food safety and public health [1]. Antibiotic resistance has been identified as a main public health concern by the World Health Organization [2, 3]. Antibiotics are most common strategy used in the treatment of bacterial infections, in addition, antibacterial metals are widely used to prevent bacterial attachment and to combat biofilms in hospital and food processing settings [2].

Antibiotics have been detected in sewage effluents, ground and surface water, sewage sludge, soil, and manure. Studies on the fate of antibiotics are motivated by two main concerns; first, antibiotics in the environment may contribute to the development of antibiotic resistant pathogens, second, the ecological consequences of antibiotic contamination that may enter in the human food chain. In a study conducted by Clarke and Smith on antibiotics in biosolids, norfloxacin, ofloxacin, ciprofloxacin, and doxycycline were measured in the sludge of a Swedish WWTP. Similar concentrations of ciprofloxacin and norfloxacin were also observed in sewage sludge samples from Switzerland. The concentration of these antibiotics was at the low mg $kg^{-1}$ dry weight range and was constant during the treatment processes. The same compounds and concentration were measured in soil that was amended by biosolids. Some of the compounds, for instance, carbamazepine and sulfamethazine can be translocated from the soil into the aerial plant components by uptake mechanisms in greenhouse plants [4].

Kim and Aga [5] studied the effects of antibiotics and ARB of wastewater treatment plants (WWTPs) on ecology and human health. Their study introduced the WWTPs as a point contamination source of persistent pharmaceuticals that affect the design and operation of treatment systems, antibiotic resistance development among pathogenic bacteria, and accumulation of persistent pharmaceuticals in soil and water. Their study estimated concentrations of antibiotics in untreated municipal wastewater in the United States and showed their possible metabolites in activated sludge [5]. They concluded that the disappearance of the parent pharmaceuticals in WWTPs does not certainly mean their complete removal. The presence of pharmaceuticals in the aquatic environment has ecotoxicological effects that impact the algal community structure and shifts the food web structure of streams [5]. The potential ecological and health impacts of antibiotics in the environment were investigated using environmental risk assessment including a two-stage process; estimation of expected introductory concentration (EIC) entering the environment and predicted environmental concentration (PEC). PEC is needed if the drug has the potential to bioaccumulate in the environment [5].

Determination and characterization of pharmaceutical compounds, antibiotics in particular, has attracted attention because of their ecotoxicological effects [5–7]. Antibiotics, such as tetracycline, sulfamethoxazole, ciprofloxacin, norfloxacin, trimethoprim, and ofloxacin, are determined in high concentration in the sludge of different WWTPs. In a study directed by Martin [6] sludge from four sludge stabilization treatments including anaerobic digestion, aerobic digestion, composting and the lagoon was monitored to detect the occurrence of 22 pharmaceutically active compounds. The average concentrations of studied compounds were 179, 310 and 142 μg/kg of sludge dry matter in primary sludge, secondary sludge, and mixed sludge, respectively. Sewage sludge that is used for the land application is always treated during one or more treatment processes namely, lime stabilization, thickening, dewatering, drying, anaerobic digestion or composting processes. However, many contaminants like antibiotic compounds may not be removed efficiently [6].

There is a report on the presence of 24 pharmaceuticals in 12 municipal and 4 livestock wastewater sludge showing that 17 and 14 pharmaceuticals were presented in municipal and livestock WWTPs, respectively. Nonsteroidal anti-inflammatory drugs were dominant in municipal WWTPs ranging from 0.42 to 367 mg/kg, whereas antibiotics (43.6 to 142 mg/kg) were dominant in livestock WWTPs [7]. The wide use of antibiotics in the livestock industry resulted in resistance of antibiotics to degradation that can lead to antibiotic resistance development in the environment [7].

The concentration of 16 antibiotics was measured in sewage and activated sludge samples using high-performance liquid chromatography-tandem mass spectrometry [8]. Statistical analysis included general analysis (averages and standard errors), cluster analysis, and correlation and regression analysis (Pearson analysis). Their study found significant correlations between the relative abundance of ARGs and the corresponding residual antibiotic concentrations and heavy metals in the effluents of WWTPs and pre-treatment units for the antibiotics or metals are suggested. Further studies are essential to prove the causation of the results of this study [8].

## 2. Occurrence of antibiotic resistance in WWTPs

High concentration of antibiotics and their associated ARB and ARGs in the effluent of WWTPs enter the environment through WWTPs discharges to rivers, wastewater reuse, irrigation and amending the soil by biosolids make. Antibiotic resistance genes can persist in the environment even when there is no antibiotic pressure.

Du et al. [9] studied ARGs including *tet(X)*, *tet*(*W*), *tet(G)*, *sul(1)*, and *intI(1)* in the influent and effluent of different units of a municipal WWTP. The studied plant possessed the anaerobic/anoxic/aerobic membrane bioreactors (MBR). The decrease of ARGs in anaerobic and anoxic units followed by an increase of ARGs in aerobic units and then decline of ARGs in MBR units was reported in this study [9]. Anaerobic and anoxic treatments methods were more effective than aerobic treatment methods at removing ARGs. Because microorganisms have lower bioactivity under anaerobic condition and the propagation of resistance genes are inhibited [9]. Furthermore, a significant positive correlation was observed between ARGs and 16S rDNA in the wastewater treatment process [9].

Wang et al. [10] conducted a study to explore the concentration of five tetracyclines, four sulfonamides, and six fluoroquinolones in the rhizosphere soil that was irrigated by reclaimed wastewater for a long time. The total concentration of tetracycline was in the range of 12.7–145.2 μg $kg^{-1}$ while no sulfonamide was found in samples. Fluoroquinolones were randomly detected in soils and their highest total concentration was 79.2 μg $kg^{-1}$. Based on the results of this study, soils that are irrigated by reclaimed wastewater accumulate antibiotics in several folds higher concentrations compared to the antibiotic concentration in the wastewater [10].

Wang and his research group studied soils of six public parks which were irrigated by the reclaimed wastewater. There was no antibiotic pressure but sulfonamide resistance genes (*sul(1)* and *sul(2)*) persisted in the soil. This result indicated that ARGs are more permanent

| Treatment Method | Target | Biosolid (copies/mL) | Effluent (copies/mL) | Reference |
|---|---|---|---|---|
| Activated sludge | *tetO, tetW, sul1* | $1.00 \times 10^8$–$1.78 \times 10^9$ | $9.12 \times 10^5$–$1.05 \times 10^6$ | [12] |
| Activated sludge | *tetC* | $3.09 \times 10^8$–$9.33 \times 10^8$ | ND* – $1.32 \times 10^4$ | [13] |
| chlorination | *tetA* | $1.23 \times 10^8$–$1.29 \times 10^9$ | ND – $2.14 \times 10^4$ | |
| Activated sludge and chlorination and UV | *tetQ* | $2.51 \times 10^8$–$10^9$ | $6.31 \times 10^3$–$1.58 \times 10^6$ | [14] |
| | *tetG* | $3.16 \times 10^8$–$1.58 \times 10^9$ | $1.58 \times 10^4$–$7.94 \times 10^5$ | |
| Activated sludge and chlorination | *tetO* | $9.7 \times 10^4$ | $2.5 \times 10^2$ | [15] |
| | *tetQ* | $8.7 \times 10^4$ | $1.6 \times 10^2$ | |
| | *tetW* | $1.8 \times 10^5$ | $4.4 \times 10^2$ | |
| | *tetH* | $5.6 \times 10^4$ | $1.6 \times 10^1$ | |
| | *tetZ* | $2.2 \times 10^5$ | $5.5 \times 10^3$ | |
| Different WWTPs | *tetW* | $9.53 \times 10^8$ | — | [16] |
| | *tetO* | $3.15 \times 10^8$ | | |
| | *sul1* | $6.04 \times 10^8$ | | |
| Conventional | *tetW* | $2.34 \times 10^5$–$2.51 \times 10^7$ | ND – $4.27 \times 10^3$ | [17] |
| | *tetO* | $6.31 \times 10^6$–$1.74 \times 10^9$ | ND – $9.12 \times 10^3$ | |
| | *sul1* | $5.62 \times 10^6$–$2.51 \times 10^9$ | $2.34 \times 10^4$–$5.62 \times 10^6$ | |

*ND = nondetectable.

**Table 1.** Results of studies on ARGs concentrations (tetracycline and sulfonamide) in WWTPs.

rather than antibiotics [10]. Based on the results of a study on removal of ARB and ARGs from urban wastewater, the abundance of 16S rRNA, *intI1, sul(1), qnrS*, $bla_{CTX-M}$, and $bla_{TEM}$ was increased to pre-treatment amount after 3 days of storage of treated wastewater [11]. Hence, it is important to find effective processes to prevent bacterial reactivation before discharge or reuse of wastewater. **Table 1** is reporting concentrations of ARGs in samples from biosolid and effluent of different WWTPs.

### 2.1. Effect of metal on ARGs development at WWTPs

The world is getting progressively more industrialized and urbanized which leads to elevation of heavy metals concentrations into the environment. Human activities such as mining, waste disposal, and corrosion of metals introduce more metal contaminations into the environment [18]. Population growth and industrial development have resulted in the increase in the discharge of industrial effluents in the environment. The effluent contains antibiotics and heavy metals which can trigger antibiotic- and heavy metal- resistance. ARB and heavy metal resistant bacteria and their associated genes are a public health concern.

Municipal wastewater is a hotspot for emerging contaminants namely antibiotics, heavy metals, ARGs, and heavy metal resistance genes (HMRGs). There are bacteria like *Escherichia coli* and *Salmonella* that are resistant to multiple antibiotics and heavy metal [19]. There is some experimental evidence showing a relation between the acquisition of HMRGs and ARGs by the mechanism of co-selection [20, 21].

Genetic co-selection of resistance genes occurs when in the presence of a stress, the selection of the associated resistance gene results in the persistence of additional resistance genes [20, 22]. Co-selection happens even without a straight effect of their specific stressors. Antibiotics and metals, as sources of environmental stresses, can affect bacterial antibiotic susceptibility and heavy metal resistance promotion. Regularly the presence of mobile genetic elements (MGEs) carrying multiple resistant genes results in co-selection [20, 23]. The molecular mechanisms behind the development of heavy metal resistance are almost similar to mechanisms which explain antibiotic resistance like efflux, by which MGEs transfer genes [23].

There are several studies investigating the common structural and functional characteristics of antibiotic-resistance and metal-resistance systems. Antibiotics namely, chloramphenicol, ciprofloxacin, coumermycin, rifampicin, tetracycline, and trimethoprim and also metals like As, Cu, Zn, Mn, Co, Ag, Hg, Cd, and Ni have been studied [21].

In another study, low total metal levels correlate with ARG abundance in soils, implying that low metal levels may co-select for antibiotic resistance [24]. In this study, the abundance of 11 ARGs was quantified by quantitative polymerase chain reaction (qPCR) assay and compared with the metal levels in the selected soils. Copper, chromium, nickel, lead, and iron significantly correlated with the abundance of ARGs [24].

Icgen and Yilmaz [19] conducted a research on the Kızılırmak River which receives industrial discharges to study co-occurrence of heavy metal and antibiotic resistance in bacteria. Twenty-four isolates were found resistant to both heavy metal and antibiotics. Resistance to heavy metals involving lead, tin, nickel, barium, aluminum, strontium, silver and lithium ranged from 50 to 92% and more than 50% of the isolates were resistant to cephalosporin, quinolone, sulfonamide and aminoglycoside classes of antibiotics. Therefore, the discharge of antimicrobials to surface water may result in co-selection of heavy metal- and antibiotic-resistant bacteria [19]. The level of heavy metal in the river varied directly with changes in industrial discharge and rainfall. The relation between heavy metal exposure level and metal- and antibiotic-resistance was not clarified.

Antibacterial properties of heavy metals may contribute to development of resistance. Antibacterial properties of nine pure metals including titanium, cobalt, nickel, copper, zinc, zirconium, molybdenum, tin, and lead have been studied using two bacterial strains, Gram-positive *Staphylococcus aureus* and Gram-negative *Escherichia coli* [25]. Based on the results, the antibacterial properties of various metals were different and among the tested metals, titanium and tin did not exhibit antibacterial properties [25]. Among the nine mentioned metals, copper and zinc are common metals in WWTPs [26–28] which are in contact with ARGs and HMRGs. Following paragraphs explain ARGs and HMRGs correlation in detail.

#### *2.1.1. Resistance mechanism acting on both metals and antibiotics*

High concentrations of anthropogenic metal contamination in the environment can apply co-selection pressure and result in antibiotic-resistance through genetic couplings [28].

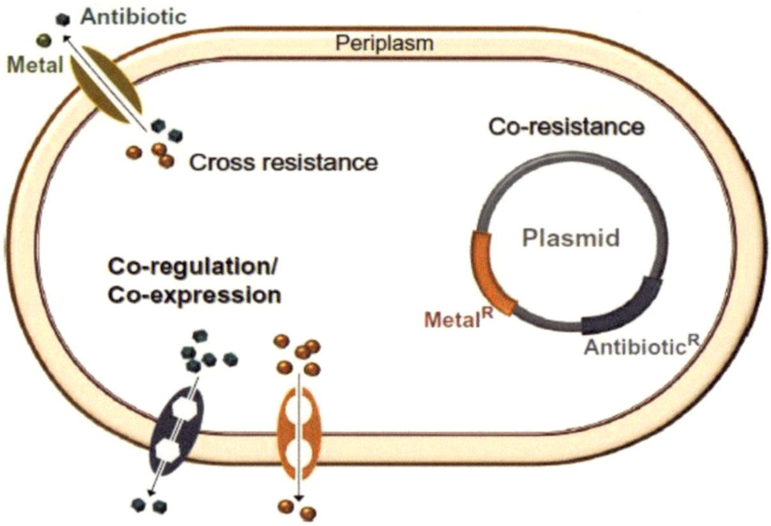


**Figure 1.** Mechanisms of co-occurrence of metal and antibiotic resistance [2].

Co-resistance, co-regulation, and cross-resistance are mechanisms of co-selection. As shown in **Figure 1**, a close linkage between two or more diverse resistance genes is called co-resistance and is known as a mechanism of antibiotic-metal co-selection [21, 29]. It seems that co-regulation can be a mechanism of antibiotic-resistance at which a number of transcriptional and translational responses to metal or antibiotic contact connected together to respond to both stresses [29]. Cross-resistance provides resistance to more than one antimicrobial agent like antibiotics and heavy metals [29].

There is a growing evidence of antibiotic resistance development derived from metal exposure. It seems that bacteria that are exposed to metals, like Cu and Zn, become resistant to metal and antibiotics simultaneously due to the metal selection of genetic elements that harbor both metal and antibiotic resistance genes [30]. There are many classes of antibiotics that can form complexes with metals and produced complexes can possess an enhanced or decayed antibiotic activity [30].

Di Cesare and his research group measured six ARGs (*tetA, sul(2),* $bla_{TEM}$, $bla_{CTX\text{-}M}$, *ermB,* and *qnrS*), two HMRGs (*czcA* and *arsB*), and the class I integron (*int1*) in different phases of three WWTPs. In their research, all the variables were classified into two groups; the first including *tetA, ermB, qnrS,* and the biotic and abiotic factors, and a second group was the genes *sul2, czcA, arsB,* and *int1*. In addition, the dynamics of *sul(2),* HMRGs, and *int1* correlated strongly. Based on this study, there is a possible relation between heavy metal contamination as well as HMRGs and spread of ARGs [20].

### *2.1.2. Environmental impacts of antibiotic and heavy metal resistance genes*

When a bacterial community is exposed to heavy metal as a selective pressure in WWTP the potential co-selection of resistant genes is very high [20]. Studies on genes encoding for resistance against different metals and of ARGs in plasmids and integrons demonstrated that these genes originate from WWTPs or soils contaminated by wastewater. The class 1 integrons, specifically, are frequently associated with gene cassettes in which both HMRGs and ARGs are present and can play an important role in co-selection mechanisms [20, 25, 30].

The effluent of WWTPs contains ARGs and HMRGs which discharges to the aquatic environment, results in the spread of ARGs and increasing the risk of gene transfer to human and animal pathogens through food chains or drinking water [1, 31]. These risks require further attention and consideration while WWTP effluents are reused as irrigation water [32].

However, the idea of co-selection of ARGs and HMRGs is supported by some studies, there is a lack of data determining the exposure level to antimicrobial metals on the selection of resistance genes.

### 2.2. Co-occurrence of antibiotic and heavy metal resistance

The results of a study on the effect of Ni, Cu, Zn, Cd, and Pb on fate and distribution of ARGs, showed a positive correlation between individual ARG and HMRGs. This result implies that heavy metals act as selective stressors and lead to the co-selection mechanism between specific metal and antibiotic resistance [1]. In their study, the abundance of *sul(3), tetA, tetM, qepA,* and *qnrA* genes had a positive correlation with Cu, Zn and Hg concentration [1].

Cu or Zn are selectors of exact bacterial populations flourishing in wastewater. Zn or Cu selected for populations of *Betaproteobacteria* and *Flavobacteria* that result in multidrug resistance against carbapenems and third-generation cephalosporins [31]. Based on the review of different studies on ARGs development in WWTP, Cu, Zn are common and in high concentration in the municipal wastewater [1, 26–28, 33–35].

Baker-Austin et al. [21] studied experimental evidence presenting a relation between HMRGs and ARGs. When the genes corresponding to resistant phenotypes are on the same genetic element (plasmid, transposon or integron) co-selection occurs, and this physical relation leads to the co-selection for other genes located on the same element [21]. The genetic traits contributed to mercury- resistance and antibiotic-resistance were established and showed that mercury- resistance was co-transferred with antibiotic resistance in a subset of mating between *Enterobacteriaceae* and recipients. There are two critical points that explain the importance of studying HMRG occurrence; co-selection mechanism and occurrence of resistance to antibacterial metals. Antibiotics namely, chloramphenicol, ciprofloxacin, coumermycin, rifampicin, tetracycline, and trimethoprim and also metals like As, Cu, Zn, Mn, Co, Ag, Hg, Cd, and Ni were studied by Baker-Austin et al. [21]. The present associations between metal contaminations and antibiotic resistance development implied the mechanisms of co-selection, including co-resistance and cross-resistance. This research group also reviewed the role of metals as a factor in co-selection and distribution of antibiotic resistance. As shown in **Table 2**, antibiotic resistance and metal resistance have common structural and functional characteristics.

Based on the literature review, there are discrepancies in our current knowledge of the dominant mechanisms of co-selection for metal- and antibiotic-resistance at the population and community level and investigation of whether metals maintain a pool of horizontally transferable antibiotic-resistance determinants.

| Resistance mechanism | Metal ions | Antibiotics |
|---|---|---|
| Reduction in permeability | As, Cu, Zn, Mn, Co, Ag | Cip, Tet, Chlor, ß-lactams |
| Drug and metal alterations | As, Hg | ß-lactams, Chlor |
| Drug and metal efflux | Cu, Co, Zn, Cd, Ni, As | Tet, Chlor, ß-lactams |
| Alteration of cellular targets | Hg, Zn, Cu | Cip, ß-lactams, Trim, Rif |
| Drug and metal sequestration | Zn, Cd, Cu | CouA |

**Table 2.** Shared characteristics of antibiotic and metal resistance systems [21].

# 3. Role of WWTP in dissemination of ARG

Freshwater resources are too limited and meeting the needs for water is challenging in the last decades as urban water shortages increase [36–38]. Based on the united nations world water development report of UNESCO in 2015, up to 70% of the fresh water, we take from rivers and groundwater is devoted to irrigation [38]. The predicted increase in the global human population to 9.7 billion in 2050 will lead to an increase in water requirement for agricultural and food production purposes [39]. Hence, the reuse of treated wastewater in agriculture seems to be a practical solution for water shortage [35]. In addition, it can help freshwater ecosystems by reducing the discharge of effluent from wastewater treatment plants (WWTPs) and preventing eutrophication and algal blooms [35].

Treated urban wastewater contains organic substances (e.g., antibiotics) and inorganic matters including pathogens, ARB and ARGs [40]. The reuse of treated wastewater may result in contamination of the environment and spread of ARB and ARGs and trigger public health concerns. One of the applications of treated wastewater is irrigation which is encouraged by governments and official organization especially because of water shortage and poverty in developing countries and urban areas [36, 41–43].

Zhang et al. [43] studied the contribution of wastewater treatment to the antibiotic resistance development of *Acinetobacter* spp. that are found in many environments, including water, soil, sewage, and food. In this study, *Acinetobacter* spp. isolates from five different sites including raw influent, second effluent, and final effluent of WWTP and upstream and downstream of the treated wastewater discharge point. This study determined the antibiotic susceptibility phenotypes using the disc-diffusion method for eight antibiotics that includes amoxicillin, chloramphenicol, ciprofloxacin, colistin, gentamicin, rifampin, sulfisoxazole, and trimethoprim. This research concluded that conventional biological treatment process in WWTPs increases the ARB population [43].

Another comprehensive study detected 140 plasmid-borne ARGs of the WWTP using polymerase chain reaction (PCR) method [44]. In this study, 192 resistance-gene-specific PCR primer pairs were designed and synthesized. Samples were collected from activated sludge and the final effluents of the WWTP. The methods included (a) isolation of plasmids from resistant bacteria, (b) selection of target reference ARGs and design of PCR primers, (c) PCR and amplicon detection, (d) sequencing and analysis of selected resistance-gene-specific amplicons. Based on the results of this study, bacteria of the WWTP share a mobile pool of ARGs that result in genetic exchange between clinical and WWTP bacteria. The final effluent of WWTP also contained ARB that confirms that the WWTP's final effluents are disseminating antibiotic resistance in the environment [44].

Recently, Zhang et al. studied both cell-free DNA and cell-associated DNA as a source for ARGs that are related to WWTPs. The cell-free DNA is extracellular DNA that can transform into other cells, and cell-associated DNA is intercellular DNA. The 0.22 μm filter intercepts intercellular DNA and extracellular DNA (filtrates contains the extracellular DNA). In this research, four ARGs (*sul(2), tet(C),* $bla_{PSE-1}$, and *erm(B)*) as cell-associated and cell-free fractions were studied. The cell-associated DNA and cell-free DNA were independently extracted and ARGs copy numbers were quantified using qPCR. Based on the results of this study, cell-associated ARGs were more than ARGs fraction in the raw wastewater, however, after biological treatment, sludge settling, membrane filtration, and disinfection, cell-associated ARGs were removed considerably and cell-free ARGs removal was much lower. Therefore, the abundance ratio of cell-free ARGs to cell-associated ARGs increased. Cell-free ARGs are important pollutants from WWTPs which are potential risks to the effluent receiving environments [45].

Munir and Xagoraraki [16] quantified 18 biosolids samples from seven WWTPs using qPCR methods. The mean concentrations of *tet(W), tet(O),* and *sul(1)* in all samples of biosolids were $9.53 \times 10^8$, $3.15 \times 10^8$, and $6.04 \times 10^8$, respectively. Lime-stabilized biosolids had considerably ($p < 0.05$) lower concentrations of ARGs compared with other biosolids treatment methods. In this study, two different sites were observed for 4 months to investigate levels of ARGs (*tet(W), tet(O),* and *sul(1)*) in soils fertilized with manure or biosolids. The concentration of ARGs was higher in manure than biosolids, but surprisingly, the results showed no notable change in the concentration of ARGs in the samples of soil, since genetic diversity and natural characteristics of background soil minimized the effect of biosolids [16].

In a recent study by D'Angelo [46] on the potential risks of the presence of antibiotic in biosolid amendments, sorption and desorption of tetracycline were indicated. Their research was on four types of amendments including biosolids, poultry manure, wood chip litter, and rice hull litter at different temperatures. The sorption and desorption equilibrium constant in municipal biosolids was 20 times higher than other amendments since the concentration of bound $Al^{3+}$ and $Fe^{3+}$ is higher in municipal biosolids. Results showed that the sorption of tetracycline was significantly increased after treatment with alum and treatment of amendments would effectively reduce antibiotic diffusion rates [46].

The effect of treated urban wastewater irrigation on fungi diversity and soil microbial activities was studied by Alguacil and her team, in Spain. Based on this study, fungi diversity was higher in soil irrigated by fresh water, but microbial activities of soil irrigated by wastewater were much more than the soil irrigated by fresh water. Hence, wastewater not only had no negative effects on crop vitality but also developed fertility of the soil. Microbiological components are biotic factors of soil that might be altered by the increase of soil microbial biomass due to wastewater irrigation [47].

As mentioned before, WWTPs are known as sources of antibiotic resistance. Auerbach et al. [14] studied two activated sludge wastewater treatment plants and two freshwater lakes for the presence of 10 tetracycline resistance genes. Qualitative PCR and quantitative PCR methods were used to detect tetracycline resistance genes and quantify the number of tetracycline resistance gene copies per volume of sample, respectively. Their results showed that both WWTPs contain more diverse types of tetracycline resistant genes than the background natural lake water samples. They revealed that the WWTPs are a source of ARGs dissemination. *tetQ* and *tetG* in the treatment processes were attenuated, however, the UV disinfection did not reduce the ARGs [14].

Presence of specific genes encoding resistance to tetracyclines (*tetQ* [48], *tetA* [49], and *tetO* [50]), sulfonamide (*sul*1 [49] *sul*2 [50]), erythromycin (*mphB* [49]), quinolone (*qnrD* [49] and *qnrS* [50]), beta-lactams (*cepA, cfxA* [48], $bla_{CTX-M}$, and $bla_{TEM}$ [50]), erythromycin (*ermB*), methicillin (*mecA*), vancomycin (*vanA)* [50], and aminoglycoside (*aac(3)-II, aacA4, aadA, aadB, aadE, aphA1, aphA2, strA* and *strB* [51]) were analyzed and confirmed by recent studies. The results of these studies prove that WWTPs are the main source of antibiotic resistance transmission.

## 4. Removal of ARGs and ARB by WWTPs

The effluent of WWTPs is an important source of pollution to the nation's water resources, and 3.5 million Americans annually are getting sick after touching water they thought was safe [52]. WWTPs are hotspots for emerging contaminants namely antibiotics, heavy metals, ARGs, and HMRGs [32]. Research on the related topic has shown the proliferation of ARGs [8], the occurrence of antibiotics and ARGs and their influence on the receiving river [53], and distribution of antibiotic resistance in the effluents of WWTPs [32]. In order to limit the occurrence and spread of antibiotic resistance, treatment methods should be able to destroy ARGs in addition to inactivating pathogens [54].

*Anaerobic, anoxic, and aerobic reactors* were studied to treat wastewaters contaminated by high concentrations of various ARGs [9]. Aerobic and anaerobic treatment processes are low energy and environmentally friendly strategies which are mostly used to treat chemical oxygen demand (COD); moreover, they can successfully remove ARB and ARGs [55].

The aerobic treatment happens in the presence of air and microorganisms which utilize oxygen to change over organic contaminants to carbon dioxide, water, and biomass (aerobes). The anaerobic treatment forms occur in the absence of air and anaerobes microorganisms which do not require air to change over organic contaminants to methane and carbon dioxide gas and biomass [51].

Another low energy treatment alternative is anaerobic-aerobic sequence (AAS) bioreactor that reduce carbon amount as a pretreatment in an anaerobic condition and after that perform aerobic treatment [55]. Metagenomics investigations of this treatment technique demonstrated the impact of this approach on antibiotic resistance and ARGs. AAS expelled over 85% of ARGs in the influent wastewater which implies it was more proficient than aerobic and anaerobic units (83 and 62%, respectively) [55].

In another study, Munir et al. [56] investigated the occurrence and distribution of ARGs including *sul*(1), *tet*(W), and *tet*(O) and their associated bacteria in the effluent of five WWTPs to assess the efficiency of different processes. ARGs and ARB removal ranged 2.37-log to 4.56-log in activated sludge, oxidative ditch and rotatory biological contactors and 2.57-log to 7.06-log in MBR [56].

Removal of antibiotics including sulfamethazine, sulfamethoxazole, trimethoprim, and lincomycin had been studied in five different WWTPs using aerobic/anaerobic treatment methods [57]. The results of this study showed the range of −11.2% to 69.0% efficiency for different pharmaceutical compounds including sulfamethazine, sulfamethoxazole, trimethoprim, and lincomycin. The negative removal efficiency belonged to lincomycin and because of its high load in wastewater [57].

To sum it up, aerobic reactors alone are not very effective and biological treatment methods can remove antibiotics, ARB, and ARGs successfully if anaerobic and aerobic reactors operate in sequence. Despite the fact that anaerobic treatment is energy efficient and has high performance, aerobic treatment is more common in municipal WWTPs. Anaerobic treatments are often used to treat wastewater that contains high loads of organic matter like industrial wastewater and needs warm temperature (35°C). Activated sludge, which is an aerobic treatment, is studied in this project and the results will help to advance the efficiency of activated sludge bioreactors in treatment plants.

Some studies aimed to remove ARGs in raw domestic wastewater by *constructed wetlands* with different flow configurations or plant species [58]. In addition, disinfection methods including chlorination, ultraviolet (UV) irradiation and sequential UV/chlorination treatment on the inactivation of ARGs have been studied [54, 59, 60]. Recently, nanomaterials with antimicrobial activity have been offered as a novel defense against ARGs [61]. Moreover, the removal of ARGs from treated wastewater in the coagulation process was examined [62]. In one of the recent works, the effect of biochar amendment on soil ARGs was assessed and the outcomes showed that biochar is pretty operational [63].

Many diverse combinations of *nanomaterial* have proved that antimicrobial nanotechnology can be effective defenses against drug-resistant organisms, ARB, and ARGs. Two different mechanisms are probable when nanoparticles treat antibiotic resistance; the first mechanism is called Trojan Horse that develops drug-delivery characteristics. In this system, a functionalized nanomaterial is joined with antibiotics and nanomaterial enters inside cells and afterward discharge significant amounts of toxic ions [57]. In the second system, a mix of antibiotic and nanomaterials result in synergistic impacts, that means they battle ARGs independently [61]. Meanwhile, removal efficiency and mechanism of four ARGs including *tetA*, *sul2*, *ermB*, and *ampC* have been found using graphene oxide nanosheet. The removal efficiency was reported in the range of 2.88 to 3.11 logs at 300 μg/mL nanosheet solution showing the potential of graphene oxide nanosheet as an innovative and effective adsorbent for treatment of ARGs [64].

The potential for antimicrobial nanomaterials to restrict the propagation of multi-drug resistant pathogens while avoiding the generation of new nanomaterial-resistant organisms was studied by a group of researchers led by Aruguete [61]. They prepared a combination of nanomaterials functionalized with molecular antibiotics. This combination consisted of liposomes, dendrimers, and an antibiotic that is inside of a polymer nanoparticles capsules, and inorganic nanoparticles with antibiotic molecules attached to the surfaces [61]. In this study, silver nanoparticles coated with a water-soluble polymer called polyvinylpyrrolidone were used to combat nanomaterial-resistant organisms [61]. This experiment proved that nanomaterial combinations are able to perform like an antibiotic and to be toxic to *Pseudomonas aeruginosa* bacteria which was resistant to multiple drugs [61]. The results of this study are in line with the previous reports on the silver-based polymers used as antimicrobial biomaterials for water treatment [65, 66].

Nanomaterials have been considered as a defense against multiple drug resistance because of their antimicrobial activity [59, 61, 62, 67]. Antibacterial activities of nanoparticles depend on two fundamental elements, physicochemical properties of nanoparticles and type of target bacteria. Regardless of the fact that there is a correlation in a couple of aspects of the antibacterial activity of nanoparticles, singular investigations are challenging to generalize since most of the researchers perform experiments using accessible nanoparticles and bacteria, rather than targeting particular and preferred nanoparticles or bacteria [68]. Nanoparticles which are utilized in lab-scale studies are not well-known and correlating them with physicochemical properties for full-scale production is not reliable.

A mix of nanomaterials and molecular antibiotics draws in much consideration recently, since they are effective in killing multi-drug resistant isolates of pathogenic bacterial species and combating an expansive range of ARB and ARGs [56, 69].

Nanomaterials play controversial roles in regard to antibiotic resistance; on one hand, as mentioned before, they have been considered as a defense against multiple drug resistance because of their antimicrobial activity, and on the other hand, they can encourage the development of antibiotic resistance in the environment [56, 70]. Overall, more information is needed concerning the mechanisms behind the antimicrobial activity of nanomaterials and their potential for influencing the development of resistance in environmental systems.

## 5. Future developments and perspectives

Antibiotic resistance development among bacteria is a challenging issue that requires improvement of next-generation treatment processes in WWTPs. The emergence of antibiotic resistance between pathogens increases the demand for effective treatment strategies. Knowledge gaps and future research needs are:

- Assessment of the effect of operating conditions (pH, free available chlorine, HRT, SRT, Biomass concentration) and environmental factors (temperature, COD, BOD, water flow on ARB and ARGs development during wastewater treatment,
- Determination of dominant mechanisms (mutation, selection, mechanisms of genetic exchange including conjugation, transduction, and transformation) of ARGs development, and
- Future studies should be done on the more extensive spectrum of ARBs and ARGs like fluoroquinolone, ertapenem, and levofloxacin resistance.

## Acknowledgements

The authors acknowledge funding support from the Department of Civil and Environmental Engineering, the University of North Carolina at Charlotte.

## Conflict of interest

The authors declare that the research was conducted in the absence of any commercial or financial relationships that could be construed as a potential conflict of interest.

## Author details

Fateme Barancheshme and Mariya Munir*

*Address all correspondence to: mmunir@uncc.edu

Department of Civil and Environmental Engineering, University of North Carolina at Charlotte, Charlotte, NC, United States

## References

[1] Xu YB et al. Distribution of tetracycline resistance genes and AmpC β-lactamase genes in representative non-urban sewage plants and correlations with treatment processes and heavy metals. Chemosphere. 2017;**170**(100):274-281

[2] Pal C et al. Metal resistance and its association with antibiotic resistance. In: Advances in Microbial Physiology. 1st ed. Elsevier Ltd; 2017. pp. 261-313

[3] Barancheshme F, Munir M. Strategies to combat antibiotic resistance in the wastewater treatment plants. Frontiers in Microbiology. Jan. 2018;**8**

[4] Clarke BO, Smith SR. Review of 'emerging' organic contaminants in biosolids and assessment of international research priorities for the agricultural use of biosolids. Environment International. 2011;**37**(1):226-247

[5] Kim S, Aga DS. Potential ecological and human health impacts of antibiotics and antibiotic-resistant bacteria from wastewater treatment plants. Journal of Toxicology and Environmental Health, Part B. Nov. 2007;**10**(8):559-573

[6] Martin J, Santos JL, Aparicio I, Alonso E. Pharmaceutically active compounds in sludge stabilization treatments: Anaerobic and aerobic digestion, wastewater stabilization ponds and composting. Science of the Total Environment. 2015;**503-504**:97-104

[7] Ekpeghere KI, Lee JW, Kim HY, Shin SK, Oh JE. Determination and characterization of pharmaceuticals in sludge from municipal and livestock wastewater treatment plants. Chemosphere. 2017;**168**:1211-1221

[8] Mao D et al. Prevalence and proliferation of antibiotic resistance genes in two municipal wastewater treatment plants. Water Research. Nov. 2015;**85**:458-466

[9] Du J, Geng J, Ren H, Ding L, Xu K, Zhang Y. Variation of antibiotic resistance genes in municipal wastewater treatment plant with A2O-MBR system. Environmental Science and Pollution Research. 2015;**22**(5):3715-3726

[10] Wang FH et al. Impact of reclaimed water irrigation on antibiotic resistance in public parks, Beijing, China. Environmental Pollution. 2014;**184**:247-253

[11] Moreira NFF et al. Solar treatment ($H_2O_2$, $TiO_2$-P25 and GO-$TiO_2$ photocatalysis, photo-Fenton) of organic micropollutants, human pathogen indicators, antibiotic resistant bacteria and related genes in urban wastewater. Water Research. May 2018;**135**:195-206

[12] Gao P, Munir M, Xagoraraki I. Correlation of tetracycline and sulfonamide antibiotics with corresponding resistance genes and resistant bacteria in a conventional municipal wastewater treatment plant. Science of the Total Environment. Apr. 2012;**421-422**:173-183

[13] Zhang T, Ming Z, XuXiang Z, HanPing F. Tetracycline resistance genes and tetracycline resistant lactose-fermenting Enterobacteriaceae in activated sludge of sewage treatment plants. Environmental Science & Technology. 2009;**43**(10):3455-3460

[14] Auerbach EA, Seyfried EE, McMahon KD. Tetracycline resistance genes in activated sludge wastewater treatment plants. Water Research. Mar. 2007;**41**(5):1143-1151

[15] Al-Jassim N, kram Ansari MI, Harb M, Hong P-YY. Removal of bacterial contaminants and antibiotic resistance genes by conventional wastewater treatment processes in Saudi Arabia: Is the treated wastewater safe to reuse for agricultural irrigation? Water Research. Apr. 2015;**73**:277-290

[16] Munir M, Xagoraraki I. Levels of antibiotic resistance genes in manure, biosolids, and fertilized soil. Journal of Environmental Quality. 2007;**40**(1):248-255

[17] Munir M, Marsh TL, Xagoraraki I. Phage metagenome and antibiotic resistance genes in sludge samples from a wastewater treatment plant. 2011;**9**(2008):2008

[18] Kang CH, So JS. Heavy metal and antibiotic resistance of ureolytic bacteria and their immobilization of heavy metals. Ecological Engineering. 2016;**97**:304-312

[19] Icgen B, Yilmaz F. Co-occurrence of antibiotic and heavy metal resistance in Kizilirmak River isolates. Bulletin of Environmental Contamination and Toxicology. 2014;**93**(6): 735-743

[20] Di Cesare A et al. Co-occurrence of integrase 1, antibiotic and heavy metal resistance genes in municipal wastewater treatment plants. Water Research. May 2016;**94**:208-214

[21] Baker-Austin C, Wright MS, Stepanauskas R, McArthur JV. Co-selection of antibiotic and metal resistance. Trends in Microbiology. Apr. 2006;**14**(4):176-182

[22] Wellington EM et al. The role of the natural environment in the emergence of antibiotic resistance in Gram-negative bacteria. The Lancet Infectious Diseases. Feb. 2013;**13**(2):155-165

[23] Yu Z, Gunn L, Wall P, Fanning S. Antimicrobial resistance and its association with tolerance to heavy metals in agriculture production. Food Microbiology. 2017;**64**:23-32

[24] Knapp CW, McCluskey SM, Singh BK, Campbell CD, Hudson G, Graham DW. Antibiotic resistance gene abundances correlate with metal and geochemical conditions in archived Scottish soils. PLoS One. Nov. 2011;**6**(11):e27300

[25] Yasuyuki M, Kunihiro K, Kurissery S, Kanavillil N, Sato Y, Kikuchi Y. Antibacterial properties of nine pure metals: A laboratory study using *Staphylococcus aureus* and *Escherichia coli*. Biofouling. 2010;**26**(7):851-858

[26] Mohammad MJ, Mazahreh N. Changes in soil fertility parameters in response to irrigation of forage crops with secondary treated wastewater. Communications in Soil Science and Plant Analysis. 2003;**34**(9-10):1281-1294

[27] Azizi S, Kamika I, Tekere M. Evaluation of heavy metal removal from wastewater in a modified packed bed biofilm reactor. PLoS One. 2016;**11**(5):1-13

[28] Li L-G, Xia Y, Zhang T. Co-occurrence of antibiotic and metal resistance genes revealed in complete genome collection. The ISME Journal. 2017;**11**(3):651-662

[29] Seiler C, Berendonk TU. Heavy metal driven co-selection of antibiotic resistance in soil and water bodies impacted by agriculture and aquaculture. Frontiers in Microbiology. 2012;**3**:1-10

[30] Poole K. At the nexus of antibiotics and metals: The impact of Cu and Zn on antibiotic activity and resistance. Trends in Microbiology. Oct. 2017;**25**(10):820-832

[31] Becerra-Castro C, Machado RA, Vaz-Moreira I, Manaia CM. Assessment of copper and zinc salts as selectors of antibiotic resistance in Gram-negative bacteria. Science of the Total Environment. Oct. 2015;**530-531**:367-372

[32] Ben W, Wang J, Cao R, Yang M, Zhang Y, Qiang Z. Distribution of antibiotic resistance in the effluents of ten municipal wastewater treatment plants in China and the effect of treatment processes. Chemosphere. 2017;**172**:392-398

[33] Aleem A, Isar J, Malik A. Impact of long-term application of industrial wastewater on the emergence of resistance traits in *Azotobacter chroococcum* isolated from rhizospheric soil. Bioresource Technology. 2003;**86**(1):7-13

[34] Jingjing Ruan YX. Stress of five heavy metals on the resistance of isolates from swine wastewater to four antibiotics. Journal of Waste Water Treatment and Analysis. 2014; **05**(03)

[35] Gatica J, Cytryn E. Impact of treated wastewater irrigation on antibiotic resistance in the soil microbiome. Environmental Science and Pollution Research. 2013;**20**(6):3529-3538

[36] Chen W, Xu J, Lu S, Jiao W, Wu L, Chang AC. Fates and transport of PPCPs in soil receiving reclaimed water irrigation. Chemosphere. 2013;**93**(10):2621-2630

[37] Alvarenga P et al. Sewage sludge, compost and other representative organic wastes as agricultural soil amendments: Benefits versus limiting factors. Waste Management. 2015;**40**(276):44-52

[38] Battude M et al. Modeling water needs and total irrigation depths of maize crop in the south west of France using high spatial and temporal resolution satellite imagery. Agricultural Water Management. 2017;**189**:123-136

[39] Hong P-Y et al. Reusing treated wastewater: Consideration of the safety aspects associated with antibiotic-resistant bacteria and antibiotic resistance genes. Water. Feb. 2018;**10**(3):244

[40] Becerra-Castro C, Lopes AR, Vaz-Moreira I, Silva EF, Manaia CM, Nunes OC. Wastewater reuse in irrigation: A microbiological perspective on implications in soil fertility and human and environmental health. Environment International. 2015;**75**:117-135

[41] SouDakouré MY, Mermoud A, Yacouba H, Boivin P. Impacts of irrigation with industrial treated wastewater on soil properties. Geoderma. 2013;**200-201**:31-39

[42] Toze S. Reuse of effluent water—Benefits and risks. Agricultural Water Management. 2006;**80**(1-3):147-159

[43] Zhang Y, Marrs CF, Simon C, Xi C. Wastewater treatment contributes to selective increase of antibiotic resistance among *Acinetobacter* spp. Science of the Total Environment. Jun. 2009;**407**(12):3702-3706

[44] Szczepanowski R et al. Detection of 140 clinically relevant antibiotic-resistance genes in the plasmid metagenome of wastewater treatment plant bacteria showing reduced susceptibility to selected antibiotics. Microbiology. Jul. 2009;**155**(7):2306-2319

[45] Zhang Y et al. Cell-free DNA: A neglected source for antibiotic resistance genes spreading from WWTPs. Environmental Science & Technology. Jan. 2018;**52**(1):248-257

[46] D'Angelo E. Sorption-desorption equilibrium and diffusion of tetracycline in poultry litter and municipal biosolids soil amendments. Chemosphere. 2017;**188**:494-501

[47] Alguacil M d M, Torrecillas E, Torres P, Garcia-Orenes F, Roldan A. Long-term effects of irrigation with waste water on soil AM fungi diversity and microbial activities: The implications for agro-ecosystem resilience. PLoS One. 2012;**7**(10):e47680

[48] Niestępski S, Harnisz M, Korzeniewska E, Osińska A. The occurrence of specific markers of *Bacteroides fragilis* group, *B. dorei* and antibiotic-resistance genes in the wastewater treatment plants. E3S Web Conference. Jul. 2018;**44**:00124

[49] Yuan Q-B, Zhai Y-F, Mao B-Y, Hu N. Antibiotic resistance genes and int I1 prevalence in a swine wastewater treatment plant and correlation with metal resistance, bacterial community and wastewater parameters. Ecotoxicology and Environmental Safety. Oct. 2018;**161**(May):251-259

[50] McConnell MM, Truelstrup Hansen L, Jamieson RC, Neudorf KD, Yost CK, Tong A. Removal of antibiotic resistance genes in two tertiary level municipal wastewater treatment plants. Science of the Total Environment. Dec. 2018;**643**:292-300

[51] Selvaraj G-K, Tian Z, Zhang H, Jayaraman M, Yang M, Zhang Y. Culture-based study on the development of antibiotic resistance in a biological wastewater system treating stepwise increasing doses of streptomycin. AMB Express. Dec. 2018;**8**(1):12

[52] American Rivers. How Sewage Pollution Ends up in Rivers. 2017. [Online]. Available: https://www.americanrivers.org/threats-solutions/clean-water/sewage-pollution/

[53] Rodriguez-Mozaz S et al. Occurrence of antibiotics and antibiotic resistance genes in hospital and urban wastewaters and their impact on the receiving river. Water Research. 2015;**69**:234-242

[54] McKinney CW, Pruden A. Ultraviolet disinfection of antibiotic resistant bacteria and their antibiotic resistance genes in water and wastewater. Environmental Science & Technology. 2012;**46**(24):13393-13400

[55] Christgen B et al. Metagenomics shows that low-energy anaerobic-aerobic treatment reactors reduce antibiotic resistance gene levels from domestic wastewater. Environmental Science & Technology. 2015;**49**(4):2577-2584

[56] Munir M, Wong K, Xagoraraki I. Release of antibiotic resistant bacteria and genes in the effluent and biosolids of five wastewater utilities in Michigan. Water Research. Jan. 2011;**45**(2):681-693

[57] Behera SK, Kim HW, Oh JE, Park HS. Occurrence and removal of antibiotics, hormones and several other pharmaceuticals in wastewater treatment plants of the largest industrial city of Korea. Science of the Total Environment. 2011;**409**(20):4351-4360

[58] Chen J et al. Removal of antibiotics and antibiotic resistance genes from domestic sewage by constructed wetlands: Effect of flow configuration and plant species. Science of the Total Environment. 2016;**571**:974-982

[59] Zhuang Y et al. Inactivation of antibiotic resistance genes in municipal wastewater by chlorination, ultraviolet, and ozonation disinfection. Environmental Science and Pollution Research. May 2015;**22**(9):7037-7044

[60] Sharma VK, Johnson N, Cizmas L, McDonald TJ, Kim H. A review of the influence of treatment strategies on antibiotic resistant bacteria and antibiotic resistance genes. Chemosphere. 2016;**150**:702-714

[61] Aruguete DM et al. Antimicrobial nanotechnology: Its potential for the effective management of microbial drug resistance and implications for research needs in microbial nanotoxicology. Environmental Science: Processes & Impacts. 2013;**15**(1):93

[62] Xiao F, Simcik MF, Gulliver JS. Mechanisms for removal of perfluorooctane sulfonate (PFOS) and perfluorooctanoate (PFOA) from drinking water by conventional and enhanced coagulation. Water Research. 2013;**47**(1):49-56

[63] Ye M et al. Effect of biochar amendment on the control of soil sulfonamides, antibiotic-resistant bacteria, and gene enrichment in lettuce tissues. Journal of Hazardous Materials. 2016;**309**:219-227

[64] Yu W, Zhan S, Shen Z, Zhou Q, Yang D. Efficient removal mechanism for antibiotic resistance genes from aquatic environments by graphene oxide nanosheet. Chemical Engineering Journal. Apr. 2017;**313**:836-846

[65] Monteiro DR, Gorup LF, Takamiya AS, Ruvollo-Filho AC, de Camargo ER, Barbosa DB. The growing importance of materials that prevent microbial adhesion: Antimicrobial effect of medical devices containing silver. International Journal of Antimicrobial Agents. 2009;**34**(2):103-110

[66] Miller JH et al. Effect of silver nanoparticles and antibiotics on antibiotic resistance genes in anaerobic digestion. Water Environment Research. May 2013;**85**(5):411-421

[67] Fang H et al. Occurrence and elimination of antibiotic resistance genes in a long-term operation integrated surface flow constructed wetland. Chemosphere. 2017;**173**:99-106

[68] Hajipour MJ et al. Antibacterial properties of nanoparticles. Trends in Biotechnology. Oct. 2012;**30**(10):499-511

[69] Shahverdi AR, Fakhimi A, Shahverdi HR, Minaian S. Synthesis and effect of silver nanoparticles on the antibacterial activity of different antibiotics against *Staphylococcus aureus* and *Escherichia coli*. Nanomedicine: Nanotechnology, Biology and Medicine. 2007;**3**(2):168-171

[70] Lam SJ et al. Combating multidrug-resistant Gram-negative bacteria with structurally nanoengineered antimicrobial peptide polymers. Nature Microbiology. Sep. 2016;**1**:16162

Chapter 6

# Multidrug Resistance in Zoonotic Pathogens: Are Medicinal Plants a Therapeuthic Alternative?

Marina Spinu, Mihaela Niculae, Silvana Popescu,
Emoke Pall and Carmen Dana Sandru

Additional information is available at the end of the chapter

http://dx.doi.org/10.5772/intechopen.81703

**Abstract**

Multidrug resistance (MDR) represents a complex phenomenon, caused not only by nondiscriminative antibiotic therapy in both human and animal medicine but also by the transfer of resistance genes between different bacteria. Animals besides different environments embody a niche for the development of resistant microbiomes, representing a serious threat to people not only as contacts but also as consumers/tourists. The epidemiological cycle of MDR bacteria is closed by changes in either their hosts or in their habitats. To prevent further spreading of MDR, natural solutions are investigated as efficacy, including in this category various compounds isolated from medicinal plants (quinones, flavones, flavonoids, and flavonols, tannins, coumarins, terpenoids and essential oils, alkaloids, lectins and polypeptides, etc.). The results of such studies are valuable for the medicine, but could the medicinal plants cover the gap for humans, animals, and the environment? This chapter aims at trying to answer this question.

**Keywords:** zoonotic bacteria, animals, multidrug resistance, medicinal plants, MIC/MBC

## 1. Introduction

Animal use paralleles, for millennia, with the development of human society; these sentient beings serve not only as working tools, weapons, and food source, but also as pets and companions. This closely interdependent and complex coexistence in a sometimes very narrow ecological niche led to an occasionally interchangeable, closely related pathology. Diseases that evolve at the level of human-animal-environment interface could negatively interfere not only with health at all levels, but also impact on economy and implicitly on welfare and social status of the population [1]. Human and animal matrices reciprocally transfer emerging or reemerging pathogens by direct contact, through food/feed and water, or sharing the habitat, and this occurrence gives rise to the so-called zoonoses [2]. A significant number of zoonotic disease are caused by bacteria, for control, treatment, and prevention of which antibiotics represented, and still represent a powerful tool. Nonetheless, antibiotic treatments, which spread exponentially, especially in preventing diseases ignoring the real infectious pressure, created a very tough, artificial selection, the survival rate of resistant bacteria becoming higher and higher [1]. One of the crucial, but sometimes disregarded sectors in generating and spreading antimicrobial resistance and increasing the public health risks is represented by animal farms, encompassing intensive raising technologies [3]. A proper understanding of the main features of this sector in segments such as the increased spreading of resistant bacteria due to the presence of a broad susceptible population, supports the disease-control strategies, management of global health risks, and improvement of health security [1]. Institutions such as World Health Organization (WHO), Food and Agriculture Organization of the United Nations (FAO), World Organization for Animal Health (OIE) co-work with international bodies, political actors, researchers, universities, and other institutions to preclude and control these hazards and the multiple impacts exerted by encouraging multiple collaborations, developing short-, mid-, and long-term strategies and efficient tools encouraging their implementation and use and also involving the relevant decision makers and stakeholders [4].

Since the discovery of penicillin by Fleming in 1928 [5], "antimicrobial" use has spread through the fields of human and animal health, to environment including various habitats and thus wildlife (**Figure 1**). Not only bacteria from the various natural animal niches became resistant, but also the antibiotic resistance was indicated in bacterioplankton [6] and proved to

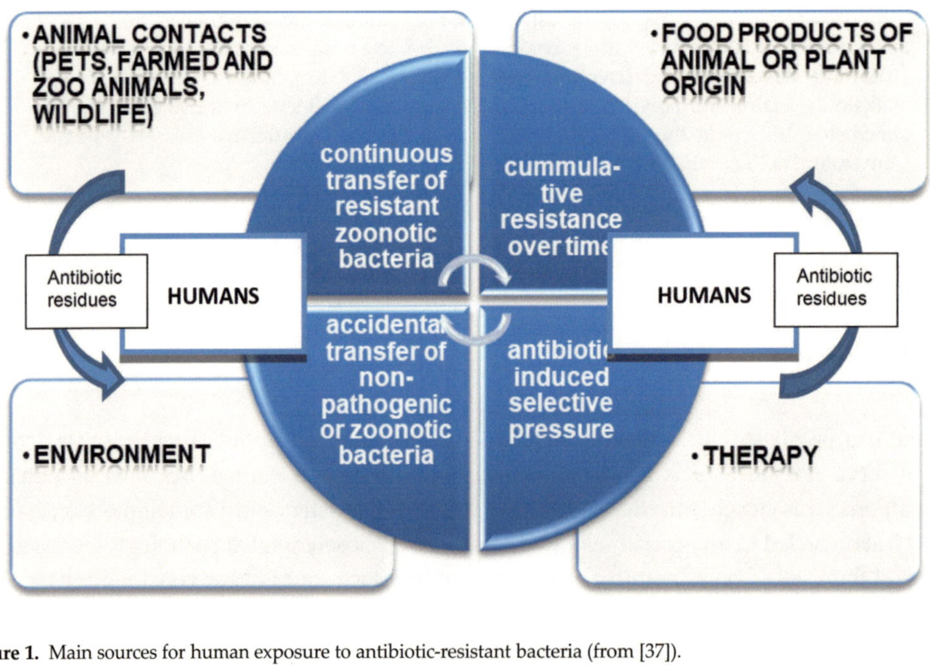


**Figure 1.** Main sources for human exposure to antibiotic-resistant bacteria (from [37]).

be dependent on geochemical conditions in the soil [7, 8]. Antibiotic resistance seems to be positively strongly correlated with the heavy metal pollution of the environment [7, 9–12].

Without a scientifically supported knowledge, vegetal extracts from various sources were used for millennia to treat infections, diminishing the negative impact of numerous bacteria. Modern medicine requires scientific evidence to support and confirm the expected therapeutic efficacy [13]; thus, the number of researches on plant extract properties augmented over the years and currently belongs to a worldwide recognized strategy aimed at identifying biologically active compounds that represent a viable alternative to synthetic drug substances demonstrated with various inconveniences (multiple side effects, nonselective toxicity, high production costs) or that have lost their initial efficacy [13]. Although different trends were described over the years, natural source importance was not minimized, as they provide key scaffolds for drug development particularly in case of antimicrobial drug development [13–19].

Briefly, the use of medicinal plants and their extracts as antimicrobials for therapy, although known for centuries, is far from being a closed subject. Medicine and biochemistry show a continuously increasing interest to this field, resulting in the introduction in practice of novel preparations, gaining new meanings within modern prophylactic and therapeutic alternatives.

Since the discovery of new molecules is apparently slower compared to bacteria resistance level increase, an integrated approach allowed the screening of various plant genera, confirmation and characterization of their antimicrobial properties (in terms of antimicrobial spectrum, minimum inhibitory concentration, minimum bactericidal concentration), identification of active compounds, and of certain mechanisms of action, which led to the expansion of the application range: therapeutic products for human health and animal health, performance enhancers or feed additives for farm animals, products for plant crop protection, food preservatives [13, 18, 20–22], etc. In the last decades, pharmacognosy studies on medicinal plants cleared numerous aspects of their bioactivity, certain ways, and sites of action of phytomedicinal compounds [23, 24]. With the progress of science and analytical laboratory methods, it has been proven that extracts from plants, containing numerous chemically active compounds such as alkaloids, tannins, polyphenols and others, could actively inhibit bacterial growth and simultaneously improve the immune response in the host by changing or inhibiting protein-protein interactions. This type of combined activity does not allow, apparently, the development of resistance [25].

Literature gathers a multitude of scientific studies that support the use of whole plant extracts in therapeutics, and the vast majority of researchers indicate medicinal plants as a viable alternative for the antimicrobials [13, 24, 26–29].

A different therapeutic approach considers plants as source for individual active compounds, not as whole extracts or solvent-based active principle mixtures. It is estimated that over 12,000 secondary plant metabolites were isolated, representing less than 10% of the total compounds found in plants. The major active molecule groups were defined as: phenolics and polyphenols, terpenoids and essential oils, alkaloids, lectins and polypeptides, polyamines, isothiocyanates, thiosulfinates, and glucosides. Nevertheless, the extraction and purification costs act as limiting for the use of individual compounds [28].

These data provide solid bases for the development of safe and effective drugs that can be used in human and veterinary medical practice [13, 30, 31].

However, mostly due to limitations associated with natural products classical screening methods, large pharmaceutical companies' interest in this category remained relatively low for several years. This particular disadvantage was significantly overcome due to the most recent strategies for natural product screening that involve an integrated multidimensional evaluation of botanical, phytochemical, and biochemical aspects, as well as advanced methods such as metabolomics and proteomics that enable the rapid identification of new compounds and production of target molecules, respectively [32, 33].

This chapter represents an overview of the most important zoonotic bacteria in terms of complexity, diversity and antimicrobial resistance, and resumes scientific data on bioactivity of medicinal plants against multidrug-resistant zoonotic bacteria isolated from animal cases.

## 2. Zoonotic bacteria complexity and diversity

Zoonotic bacteria are among the most important causes of morbidity and mortality in human, and their importance is recognized and stated by several international and national organizations [34, 35]. Furthermore, given the abundance of scientific proof of their impact on human health, international control and prevention strategies are currently implemented worldwide. In addition, numerous retrospective and prospective studies are conducted by specialized interdisciplinary research groups in order to provide more and updated knowledge on the etiopathogenesis of both already established and emerging or reemerging diseases. The economic consequences cannot be minimized, since the international protocols involve disruptions of national, regional and global trade, and substantial losses associated with animal culling and disposal of the carcasses. To acknowledge the zoonotic importance and the economic impact, certain bacterial diseases are also listed by OIE and require official notification [34]. The most common and important bacterial diseases with confirmed zoonosis status are anthrax, brucellosis, bovine tuberculosis, campylobacteriosis, listeriosis, leptospirosis, salmonellosis, psittacosis [36–38], etc.

Starting with 2010, the WHO, FAO, and OIE identified and issued priority areas that included zoonotic diseases and underlined the need for multidisciplinary collaboration to address health threats at the human-animal-ecosystem interface under the one-health concept. The one-health concept or paradigm allows the comprehensive description of the complex epidemiology in zoonotic diseases. Among the most compelling examples of the One Health paradigm, food-animal-associated zoonoses are distinguished and are monitored worldwide. It is mostly, but not exclusively, the case of foodborne diseases, with top ranked pathogens such as *Salmonella, Escherichia coli, Campylobacter* [37, 39], etc.

*Salmonella* serovars and *Escherichia coli* pathotypes were isolated from many specimens of mammalian, avian, reptilian, and amphibian origin, fish, and insect, as well as from plants, soil, and water origin; hence, the main route of transmission involves consumption of contaminated foods of both animal and vegetal origin: poultry, beef, pork, eggs, milk, fruit, vegetables [37, 39, 40], etc.

Other pathogens' transmission is related to occupational hazards, and one of the most resourceful bacterium in this regard is represented by livestock-associated methicillin-resistant *Staphylococcus aureus* (LA-MRSA), in particular the clonal complex (CC) 398 [25, 41–43]. Its first description was based on the isolation from pigs, pig handlers, and their close contacts, followed by reports involving livestock and livestock-derived food products in several countries, particularly in regions with high-density pig farming from Europe, Canada, Asia, and the USA [25, 42, 44, 45]. Grounded on recent data, colonization of LA-MRSA among persons occupationally exposed to pigs, cattle, or poultry appears to be very frequent and risk of developing MRSA infections is relatively elevated [41, 42]. The first exposed persons are not only at the risk to develop infections, but also they presumably represent the source for LA-MRSA transmission to household members [43, 46] and other parts of the human population [41], explaining the isolation of LA-MRSA from hospitals and other healthcare facilities' environment.

A substantial scientific database was collected over decades providing relevant information on zoonotic diseases that originate from farmed or food animals [37, 38, 47], but more and more figures suggested pets and wild animals were significant sources and reservoirs of zoonotic bacteria [48–52]. Regarding pets, the great majority of the studies are focused on cats and dogs [53], but lately the range of animal species kept within households diversified to encompass rodents, rabbits, ferrets, birds, amphibians, reptiles, and ornamental fish [49]. Comparing the amount of literature data, pet-associated bacterial zoonoses are considered as a relatively neglected area compared with foodborne zoonoses [49]; thus, future studies are needed to understand the complexity of epidemiological links in these cases.

The main study approach is similar to farmed animals and targets the two main categories of sources: (1) sick animals and (2) asymptomatic carriers, considering that pets may be infected or colonized with a wide variety of bacteria pathogenic to animals and people. With respect to transmission routes, a close contact between pets and owners represents a peculiarity that suggests primarily the direct contact; petting and playing with pets along with licking or minor physical injuries (usually affecting the skin on the hands) may be associated with local or systemic pathologies especially in risk categories that include young, old, pregnant, and immunosuppression individuals. Secondly, the food, water, and the environment may be contaminated by pets' fecal and skin microbiota [54, 55].

The above-mentioned aspects are reunited due to the increasingly popular trend of feeding raw meat-based diets (RMBDs) [56–58], with several studies underlining the serious risks to both animal and human health, given the laboratory confirmed presence of zoonotic bacteria and parasite pathogens in commercial RMBDs. Fresh, refrigerated, and frozen RMBDs may represent the source of *Escherichia coli* serotype O157:H7, extended-spectrum beta-lactamases-producing *E. coli*, *Listeria monocytogenes*, *Salmonella* species such as *S. typhimurium*, *S.* Heidelberg, and *S.* Kentucky [54, 56, 57, 59, 60]. Feces appear to represent an important source of Gram-negative bacteria with zoonotic potential, and several studies indicated a positive correlation between the raw meat feeding and *Salmonella*-active fecal shedding. Although it may not be representative for the general population of dogs, a special canine category was investigated in this regard—the case of dogs that participate in animal-assisted interventions (AAIs), also named "therapy dogs": since these animals commonly interact with immunocompromised people, the risks cannot be minimized [54, 56, 57, 61].

## 3. Multidrug resistance in animals

Antimicrobial Resistance Global Report on surveillance [62], issued in 2014 by WHO warned, based on surveillance data recorded, on the major problem represented by antibiotic resistance in a "postantibiotic era. "This definition underlined that most antibiotics, while considered a panacea, were broadly misused in both humans and food-producing animals, thus leading for widespread MDR. In parallel with the discovery of new antibacterial classes of compounds, the induction of resistance was followed closely by the drugs selecting the most resistant of the pathogens, which further spread [62].

One of the less regarded, yet significant sectors in spreading MDR, is represented by the animal segment, and little is known about the epidemiology of MDR in food animals and lesser in wildlife. Similarly to human medicine, veterinary antibiotics in use fail to control not only infections related to conventional agents but are also ubiquitous and commensal bacteria turned into aggressive pathogens. Not only antimicrobial use to control medical situations, such as herd- or flock-based infections (pneumonia, neonatal infections and infections occurring in immune-suppressed animals, surgeries, etc.) [62], but also the use of antimicrobials as growth enhancers in food-producing farmed species (poultry, swine, and cattle) increased the risk represented by animals in spreading MDR. Morbidity and mortality caused by bacteria resistant to commonly used and available for veterinary antibiotics are not the single causes for economic losses in farmed animals. Supplementary cost must be added for food control for antibiotic residues and resistant bacteria in food and disposal of contaminated items. There are many researches on the use of quantitatively active antimicrobial ingredients in farmed animals, showing the amount far exceeds that used in humans.

*Enterobacteriaceae* represent a large bacteria family, including numerous genera inhabiting human and animal gut of which some synthesize endotoxins. The best known representatives, *E. coli* and a broad variety of *Salmonella spp.*, were subject to abundant studies. Not only these, but also some other representatives of the family show MDR and also resistance to antibiotics such as last-generation beta-lactams (i.e., carbapenem) used to treat severe bacterial infections and considered to be "the last line of antibiotic defense." A smaller group of carbapenem-resistant Enterobacteriaceae (CRE) proved to be carbapenem-nonsusceptible and extended-spectrum cephalosporin resistant, and include *Escherichia coli, Enterobacter aerogenes, Enterobacter cloacae* complex, *Klebsiella pneumoniae*, or *Klebsiella oxytoca* [63]. These species are also found in animals: the *Enterobacter* complex as commensal microflora in the intestinal tracts of mammals and fish and also pathogenic for insects [64], *E. coli* in swine, dairy cows' mastitis [65, 66], *Klebsiella oxytoca* not only in bovine mastitis [67], but also in pets [68].

Multiple antibiotic-resistant bacteria emerging in dairy cows' mastitis as a result of extensive/uncontrolled drug use, biased therapy, horizontal gene transfer, and/or spontaneous genetic mutations pose an increased health risk to humans by contaminating milk and milk products. Virulence genes in connection with antimicrobial define pathogenic, but also certain commensal strains of *E. coli*, emphasizing the risks of fecal contamination of animal-derived, including milk products, as an important source for human outbreaks. Furthermore, the severeness of illness is increased in *E. coli* by the association of MDR with Shiga-like toxin (*stx1* and *stx2*) genes' presence. For example, resistance toward several active substances from commercial products recommended for bovine pathologies: penicillin-streptomycin, tetracycline, neomycin, ampicillin, and amoxicillin/clavulanic acid was found to different extents (MAR 0.2–0.80)—was found in 125 isolates sampled from healthy dairy cows. Multidrug-resistant phenotypes (resistance to more than four antimicrobials) were recorded for 12 isolates (9.6%). The molecular analysis pointed out the presence of *stx1* gene in case of 20 strains and *stx2* for 11 strains, respectively. The presence of Shiga-like toxin genes (*stx1* and *stx2*) and high MAR index highlight the risk associated with human exposure in terms of possible contamination of milk and dairy products provided by the bovine farms. These results support compulsory food hygiene and safety measures throughout the production chain, to minimize or eliminate the contamination risk for the products provided by these farms [Crisan et al., unpublished data, 2018].

A study conducted in Canada by Finley et al. [56] indicated for commercially available canine raw food diets, an overall *Salmonella* prevalence of 21%, with chicken as an ingredient for 67% of the *Salmonella*-positive diets. Eighteen distinct serotypes displaying resistance toward 12 of the 16 antimicrobials tested, and a predominant pattern of ampicillin and tetracycline resistance entitled the authors to conclude on the need for implementing regulatory guidelines for the production of these diets aimed to reduce or to eliminate the associated risks for pets and the contact people.

Also, outbreaks of human salmonellosis related to exposure to animal-derived pet treats (pig ear, beef steak patty dog, and pet treats of seafood origin) have been reported in Canada, with the laboratory confirmation of *Salmonella* contamination in case of mentioned pet treats and identification of the following serotypes: *S.* Bovismorbificans, *S.* Give, *S.* Derby, and *S.* Typhimurium var. Copenhagen. The overall prevalence of 4% was regarded as lower compared to data reported in 1999, but the isolates showed resistance to up to seven antimicrobials [56]. A significant higher prevalence with 41% (65/158) of samples found positive for *Salmonella* was reported in case of dog treats derived from pig ears and other animal parts randomly collected in USA [28].

Updates on the antimicrobial resistance trends are needed in order to select the most suitable choices for the antibacterial therapy particularly in case of methicillin-resistant *Staphylococcus aureus* (MRSA) infections. Regarded as an opportunist organism, MRSA is responsible not only for localized skin and soft-tissue infections, but also for invasive forms such as septicemia and toxic shock syndrome [45]. Severe clinical outcomes and added costs justify further research for alternative treatments.

Due to the high diversity of MDR bacteria isolated from numerous animal sources and food of animal origin, an integrated meta-analysis of data could support the upgraded short-, medium-, and long-term strategies to control antimicrobial resistance and its further development, which in their turn are important for preventing the emergence and cross-country/continent spreading of resistant strains [69].

## 4. Medicinal plants as antibacterial agents

Numerous researchers studied the healing effects of plants and their extracts along with their beneficial effects in healthy organisms. Nowadays, plant-based therapy benefits of solid scientific support the individual chemical components or their combinations showing antimicrobial and anti-inflammatory activity, immune-stimulating potential, or anticancer effects. Since prevention is the key to good health, the researchers investigated the possibilities of using vegetal preparations to preserve health: (a) indirectly, by stimulating both innate and the adaptive immune response to antigens of various kinds and also (b) directly, by exerting either a bacteriostatic or preferably a bactericidal effect [70].

Apparently simple, the selection of plants or their extracts to be used for specific therapeutic purposes embodies the involvement of numerous factors, from health to economic impacts (**Figure 2**).

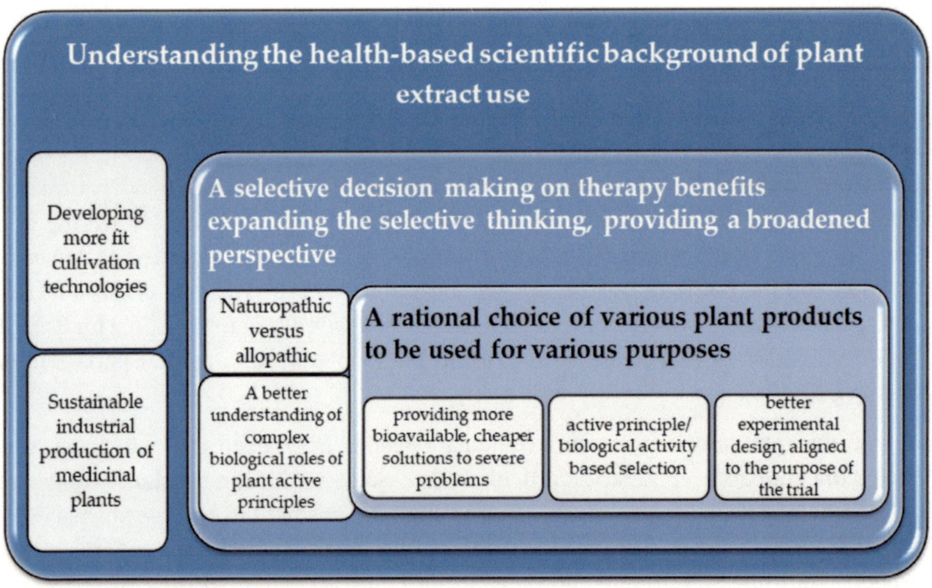


**Figure 2.** Different steps of the decision-making process in plant extract use for therapy.

### 4.1. Plant extracts acting against bacteria indirectly: immunological uses

Current trends in medicine tend to include natural products in therapy, without mixing allopathic and homeopathic treatments, the latest gaining more and more in comparison with chemically obtained compounds. The WHO list of 252 basic and essential drugs includes 11% of medications exclusively of flowering plant origin [71].

Vegetal extracts from various plant origins are used more and more, with a favorable activity in diminishing the negative impact of numerous microbial agents or in improving the innate or acquired resistance of the body to infections [17, 18, 72].

Classical therapeutic protocols supplemented with vegetal extracts could increase the protective capacity of the individuals, by their complex action mechanisms, which stimulate immunity. This pattern is actually applied in veterinary medicine, where certain stress-induced changes, caused by intensive raising/farming of food species, could be corrected in this manner [73–76]. Moreover, active principles proved to be potent in restoring the immune reactivity in individuals with induced or innate immunosuppression [77–82].

Vaccines against bacterial diseases represent one of the most powerful tools for prevention and control. Within this framework, researches on the immune stimulating activities of vegetal extractions were successful, with obvious immune modulating effects. Due to improved bioavailability as compared to conventional drugs, combined with immune modulating potential, the question on plant extracts as potential adjuvants emerged for vaccines broadly used to prevent infectious diseases, in both humans and animals. An appropriate understanding of adjuvant potential of vegetal extracts and experimental design to investigate these possibilities would lean on a good knowledge of general action mechanisms of vaccine adjuvants.

### 4.2. Direct antibacterial activity of plant extracts

Antimicrobial effects of plant extracts on clinical isolates from farmed and pet animals and their potential use to improve health and lower the risk for humans were illustrated by experiments aiming to investigate the influence of the plant taxonomy/chemical composition on the *in vitro* bacteriostatic/bactericidal effects.

Plant extracts were initially proposed as supplementary means in combined antibiotic and natural therapies; therefore, the synergism between plant extracts and antibiotics was also observed in experimental studies. In a complex research carried out to establish the antimicrobial effect of certain plants: *Achillea millefolium* (yarrow), *Caryophyllus aromaticus* (clove), *Melissa officinalis* (lemon-balm), *Ocimum basilicum* (basil), *Psidium guajava* (guava), *Punica granatum* (pomegranate), *Rosmarinus officinalis* (rosemary), *Salvia officinalis* (sage), *Syzygium jambolanum* (jambolan), and *Thymus vulgaris* (thyme) on bacteria resistant from 1 to 18 antibiotics: amikacin, ampicillin, cephalothin, cefpirome, carbenicillin, cefoxitin, chloramphenicol, ceftriaxone, cefotaxime, erythromycin, gentamicin, kanamycin, lincomycin, methicillin, nalidixic acid, netilmicin, norfloxacin, nitrofurantoin, penicillin, piperacillin, rifampicin, sulfonamide, sulfamethoxazole, tobramycin, tetracycline, vancomycin (*Proteus spp.*, *Klebsiella pneumoniae*, *Shigella spp.*, *Pseudomonas aeruginosa*,

*Enterobacter aerogenes, Escherichia coli, Staphylococcus aureus*) and susceptible collection strains (*Staphylococcus aureus* ATCC 6538, *Salmonella choleraesuis* ATCC 10708; *Pseudomonas aeruginosa* ATCC 15442), the authors indicated that clove (*Caryophyllus aromaticus*) and jambolan (*Syzygium jambolanum*) were the strongest inhibitors (64.2 and 57.1%) of the used bacterial strains. Furthermore, their activity was the most remarkable (83.3%) against the germs resistant to antibiotics, where their synergistic activity with the antibiotics was also observed. Interestingly, plants such as sage and yarrow, well known for their antiseptic properties, showed no effect on the tested MDR bacteria. Some of the plants showed in specific cases a homeopathic-like effect, i.e., clove, jambolan, pomegranate, and thyme extracts, when used in lower concentrations but combined with ineffective antibiotics against *Pseudomonas aeruginosa* [26, 27, 29, 83, 84].

| Name | Extract type | *In vitro* efficacy against | Strain origin | Evaluation method(s) | Mechanism(s) of action | References |
|---|---|---|---|---|---|---|
| *Syzygium aromaticum* and *Cinnamomum* > *Mentha spicata* L. and *Coriandrum sativum* L. > *Allium sativum* L. and *Nigella sativa* L. | Ethanolic extracts | MDR *E. coli* | Retail chicken meat samples | Broth microdilution | Not determined | [87] |
| *Olea europaea* | Ethanolic extracts | *E. coli* O157:H7 *S. enteritidis* | Reference laboratory | Broth microdilution | Inhibition of the biofilm formation for *S. enteritidis* | [16] |
| *Origanum vulgare* > *Thymus zygis Thymus mastichina* | Essential oils | *E. coli, Salmonella essen, Salmonella enteritidis,* ETEC, *Salmonella choleraesuis, Salmonella typhimurium* | Poultry swine | Broth microdilution | Not determined | [88] |
| *Melissa officinalis* > *Thymus vulgaris* and *Salvia officinalis* | Essential oils | *Staphylococcus aureus, E. coli Salmonella Enteritidis* | Bovine | Disc diffusion broth microdilution | Not determined | [89, 90] |
| *Allium sativum* L., *Elwendia persica (Bunium persicum), Oryza sativa* L. and *Triticum aestivum* L. | Ethanolic extracts | *Staphylococcus aureus, E. coli* | Bovine | Disc diffusion broth microdilution | Not determined | [91] |
| *Achyranthes aspera* L., *Ficus carica, Malva parviflora, Vernonia species, Solanum hastifolium, Calpurnia aurea* Benth, *Nicotiana tabacum* L., *Ziziphus spina-christi, Croton macrostachyus* | Hydroalcoholic extracts | *S. aureus* | Bovine | Disc diffusion broth microdilution | Not determined | [92] |

**Table 1.** Herbal extracts demonstrated to inhibit MDR zoonotic strains of animal origin.

Other well-known plants, which share immunological activity, from *Compositae* family, were further investigated for their antibacterial effects, following the principle of "the more the merrier." Echinacea, a popular plant in human medicine for its immune-stimulating and antiviral effects, also acts as an inhibitor for both tissue and bacterial hyaluronidase. This activity was considered to hinder the development and spreading of infection from localized to generalized [23, 24].

Another plant family, the Lamiaceae, has numerous examples of species with antibacterial activity. The investigation of their antibacterial activity against MDR, extended spectrum beta-lactamase-positive (ESBL), Gram-negative clinical isolates (*A. baumannii, K. pneumoniae, E. coli, P. aeruginosa*) of ethanolic extracts of *Mentha sp., Ocimum basilicum, Plectranthus barbatus,* and *Rosmarinus officinalis,* indicated that the minimal inhibiting concentration ranged from 0.5 to 2 mg/mL, while all extracts were effective against at least two of the tested bacteria [85].

Another plant from *Lamiaceae* with a less investigated antibacterial influence was considered as a potential therapeutic resource in bovine mastitis. Mastitis, one of the most economically impacting diseases of dairy cows due to subclinical status and difficult diagnosis, is heavily treated with antibiotics, leading to MDR in the involved bacterial strains. The lesser antibiotic efficacy, therefore, demands for therapeutic alternatives. In a study on the antimicrobial effectiveness of *Melissa officinalis* on the subclinical mastitis, microbiome carried out on several Romanian dairy farms ([93]), a variety of bacteria (*S. sciuri, Shigella spp. S. lentus, Acinetobacter baumannii, Chryseomonas luteola, Enterobacter cloacae, Escherichia vulneris,* etc.) were isolated with an MAR index up to 0.8 against amoxicillin+clavulanate, amoxicillin, chloramphenicol, cefoperazone, ciprofloxacin, and oxytetracycline. The *Melissa* tincture was less effective than the same plant essential oil (11.3 $\pm$ 3.6 versus 12.3 $\pm$ 4.3 mm), but comparable to amoxicillin, amoxicillin/clavulanic acid, and was higher than cefoperazone (total resistance). The efficacy depended more on the strain than on the solvent type also suggesting a therapeutic alternative to antibiotic treatment, as mentioned in the literature [86].

Most of the studies were carried out using reference strains, especially in case of the initial screening, but more recently, such assays also include clinical strains, both antimicrobial susceptible and resistant. **Table 1** summarizes relevant data on the ability of herbal extracts to inhibit MDR zoonotic strains of animal origin.

## 5. Conclusions

In spite of extensive research carried out on healing effects of plants, antibacterial effects included, the subject is far from being closed, the high variety of plant species providing a strong support for investigation. Although numerous researchers deal with the effects of individual compound against bacteria, those extracts containing multiple active substances and exerting simultaneously antibacterial and immune-enhancing effects are favored. Veterinary and zoonotic pathology, due to the presence of MDR bacteria, could equally benefit of the discovery of plant extracts with high antibacterial potential, useable separately or in combination with otherwise inefficient classical antibacterial therapies.

## Acknowledgements

We acknowledge the financial support provided by the Romanian National Research Council of the Ministry of Education by the project PNII 61/2012 and the Hungarian Academy of Sciences for performing the research on antibiotic resistances in various environments and also plant extract effects on microbes.

## Conflict of interest

None of the authors have any existing or possible conflict of interests, including financial, personal, or any other relationships, which could influence their scientific work.

## Author details

Marina Spinu*, Mihaela Niculae, Silvana Popescu, Emoke Pall and Carmen Dana Sandru

*Address all correspondence to: marina.spinu@gmail.com

Faculty of Veterinary Medicine, University of Agricultural Sciences and Veterinary Medicine, Cluj-Napoca, Romania

## References

[1] Mayer M, Vogl CR, Amorena M, Hamburger M, Walkenhorst M. Treatment of organic livestock with medicinal plants: A systematic review of European ethnoveterinary research. Forschende Komplementärmedizin. 2014;**21**(6):375-386. DOI: 10.1159/000370216

[2] Bengis RG, Leighton FA, Fischer JR, Artois M, Mörner T, Tate CM. The role of wildlife in emerging and re-emerging zoonoses. Revue Scientifique et Technique. 2004;**23**(2):497-511. Review

[3] Aminov RI. A brief history of the antibiotic era: Lessons learned and challenges for the future. Frontiers in Microbiology. 2010;**1**:134. DOI: 10.3389/fmicb.2010.00134

[4] Kalayou S, Haileselassie M, Gebre-egziabher G, Tiku'e T, Sahle S, Taddele H, et al. In-vitro antimicrobial activity screening of some ethnoveterinary medicinal plants traditionally used against mastitis, wound and gastrointestinal tract complication in Tigray Region, Ethiopia. Asian Pacific Journal of Tropical Biomedicine. 2012;**2**(7):516-522. DOI: 10.1016/S2221-1691(12)60088-4

[5] Kawamura K, Sugawara T, Matsuo N, Hayashi K, Norizuki C, Tamai K, et al. Spread of CTX-type extended-spectrum β-lactamase-producing *Escherichia coli* isolates of epidemic

clone B2-O25-ST131 among dogs and cats in Japan. Microbial Drug Resistance. 2017;**23**(8): 1059-1066. DOI: 10.1089/mdr.2016.0246

[6] Sun Y, Gong G, Guo Y, Wang Z, Song S, Zhu B, et al. Purification, structural features and immunostimulatory activity of novel polysaccharides from *Caulerpa lentillifera*. International Journal of Biological Macromolecules. 2018;**108**:314-323. DOI: 10.1016/j.ijbiomac.2017.12.016

[7] Kokoska L, Kloucek P, Leuner O, Novy P. Plant-derived products as antibacterial and antifungal agents in human health care. Current Medicinal Chemistry. 2018. DOI: 10.2174/0929867325666180831144344

[8] White DG, Datta A, McDermott P, Friedman S, Qaiyumi S, Ayers S, et al. Antimicrobial susceptibility and genetic relatedness of Salmonella serovars isolated from animal-derived dog treats in the USA. The Journal of Antimicrobial Chemotherapy. 2003;**52**(5):860-863

[9] Belay ED, Kile JC, Hall AJ, Barton-Behravesh C, Parsons MB, Salyer SJ, et al. Zoonotic disease programs for enhancing global health security. Emerging Infectious Diseases. 2017;**23**(13). DOI: 10.3201/eid2313.170544

[10] Pintar KD, Christidis T, Thomas MK, Anderson M, Nesbitt A, Keithlin J, et al. A systematic review and meta-analysis of the *Campylobacter* spp. prevalence and concentration in household pets and petting zoo animals for use in exposure assessments. PLoS One. 2015;**10**(12): e0144976. DOI: 10.1371/journal.pone.0144976

[11] Rahman H, Khan I, Hussain A, Shahat AA, Tawab A, Qasim M, et al. *Glycyrrhiza glabra* HPLC fractions: Identification of aldehydo isoophiopogonone and liquirtigenin having activity against multidrug resistant bacteria. BMC Complementary and Alternative Medicine. 2018;**18**(1):140. DOI: 10.1186/s12906-018-2207-8

[12] Stevens MP, Humphrey TJ, Maskell DJ. Molecular insights into farm animal and zoonotic Salmonella infections. Philosophical Transactions of the Royal Society of London. Series B, Biological Sciences. 2009;**364**(1530):2709-2723. DOI: 10.1098/rstb.2009.0094. Review

[13] Stepanauskas R, Glenn TC, Jagoe CH, Tuckfield RC, Lindell AH, McArthur JV. Elevated microbial tolerance to metals and antibiotics in metal-contaminated industrial environments. Environmental Science & Technology. 2005;**39**(10):3671-3678

[14] Bhatt VD, Shah TM, Nauriyal DS, Kunjadia AP, Joshi CG. Evaluation of a topical herbal drug for its in-vivo immunomodulatory effect on cytokines production and antibacterial activity in bovine subclinical mastitis. Ayu. 2014;**35**(2):198-205. DOI: 10.4103/0974-8520

[15] Loeffler A, Pfeiffer DU, Lloyd DH, Smith H, Soares-Magalhaes R, Lindsay JA. Meticillin-resistant *Staphylococcus aureus* carriage in UK veterinary staff and owners of infected pets: New risk groups. The Journal of Hospital Infection. 2010;**74**(3):282-288. DOI: 10.1016/j.jhin.2009.09.020

[16] Luna S, Krishnasamy V, Saw L, Smith L, Wagner J, Weigand J, et al. Outbreak of *E. coli* O157: H7 infections associated with exposure to animal manure in a rural community—Arizona

and Utah, June-July 2017. Morbidity and Mortality Weekly Report. 2018;**67**(23):659-662. DOI: 10.15585/mmwr.mm6723a2

[17] Nascimento GGF, Locatelli J, Freitas PC, Silva GL. Antibacterial activity of plant extracts and phytochemicals on antibioticresistant bacteria. Brazilian Journal of Microbiology. 2000;**31**:247-256

[18] Naveed R, Hussain I, Tawab A, Tariq M, Rahman M, Hameed S, et al. Antimicrobial activity of the bioactive components of essential oils from Pakistani spices against Salmonella and other multi-drug resistant bacteria. BMC Complementary and Alternative Medicine. 2013;**13**:265. DOI: 10.1186/1472-6882-13-265

[19] Niculae M, Spînu M, Şandru D, Brudaşcă F, Cadar D, Kobolkuti L, et al. Lamiaceae essential oils and alcoholic extracts and their effects on zoonotic multidrug-resistant bacteria. Planta Medica. 2009;**75**:PJ86. DOI: 10.1055/s-0029-1234891

[20] Finley R, Reid-Smith R, Ribble C, Popa M, Vandermeer M, Aramini J. The occurrence and antimicrobial susceptibility of salmonellae isolated from commercially available canine raw food diets in three Canadian cities. Zoonoses and Public Health. 2008;**55**(8-10):462-469. DOI: 10.1111/j.1863-2378.2008.01147.x

[21] Lefebvre SL, Reid-Smith R, Boerlin P, Weese JS. Evaluation of the risks of shedding Salmonellae and other potential pathogens by therapy dogs fed raw diets in Ontario and Alberta. Zoonoses and Public Health. 2008;**55**(8-10):470-480. DOI: 10.1111/j.1863-2378.2008.01145.x

[22] Valle DL Jr, Cabrera EC, Puzon JJ, Rivera WL. Antimicrobial activities of methanol, ethanol and supercritical $CO_2$ extracts of Philippine *Piper betle* L. on clinical isolates of gram positive and gram negative bacteria with transferable multiple drug resistance. PLoS One. 2016;**11**(1):e0146349. DOI: 10.1371/journal.pone.0146349

[23] Jeśman C, Młudzik A, Cybulska M. History of antibiotics and sulphonamides discoveries. Pol Merkur Lekarski. 2011;**30**(179):320-322. [Article in Polish]

[24] Silva C, Calva E, Maloy S. One health and food-borne disease: Salmonella transmission between humans, animals, and plants. Microbiology Spectrum. 2014;**2**(1). DOI: 10.1128/microbiolspec.OH-0020-2013. Review

[25] Cowan M. Plant products as antimicrobial agents. Clinical Microbiology Reviews. 1999;**12**(4):564-582

[26] Shaheen AY, Sheikh AA, Rabbani M, Aslam A, Bibi T, Liaqat F, et al. Antibacterial activity of herbal extracts against multi-drug resistant *Escherichia coli* recovered from retail chicken meat. Pakistan Journal of Pharmaceutical Sciences. 2015;**28**(4):1295-1300

[27] Sharifi-Rad M, Mnayer D, Morais-Braga MFB, Carneiro JNP, Bezerra CF, Coutinho HDM, et al. Echinacea plants as antioxidant and antibacterial agents: From traditional medicine to biotechnological applications. Phytotherapy Research. 2018;**32**(9):1653-1663. DOI: 10.1002/ptr.6101

[28] Tayel AA, Hussein H, Sorour NM, El-Tras WF. Foodborne pathogens prevention and sensory attributes enhancement in processed cheese via flavoring with plant extracts. Journal of Food Science. 2015;**80**(12):M2886-M2891. DOI: 10.1111/1750-3841.13138

[29] Van den Eede A, Martens A, Floré K, Denis O, Gasthuys F, Haesebrouck F, et al. MRSA carriage in the equine community: An investigation of horse-caretaker couples. Veterinary Microbiology. 2013;**163**(3-4):313-318. DOI: 10.1016/j.vetmic.2012.12.038

[30] Harvey AL, Edrada-Ebel R, Quinn RJ. The re-emergence of natural products for drug discovery in the genomics era. Nature Reviews. Drug Discovery. 2015;**14**(2):111-129. DOI: 10.1038/nrd4510

[31] Singh PA, Desai SD, Singh J. A review on plant antimicrobials of past decade. Current Topics in Medicinal Chemistry. 2018;**18**(10):812-833. DOI: 10.2174/156802661866618051612 3229

[32] http://www.oie.int/animal-health-in-the-world/oie-listed-diseases-2018/

[33] Markland SM, LeStrange KJ, Sharma M, Kniel KE. Old friends in new places: Exploring the role of extraintestinal *E. coli* in intestinal disease and foodborne illness. Zoonoses and Public Health. 2015;**62**(7):491-496. DOI: 10.1111/zph.12194

[34] Huang E, Gurzau AE, Hanson BM, Kates AE, Smith TC, Pettigrew MM, et al. Detection of livestock-associated methicillin-resistant *Staphylococcus aureus* among swine workers in Romania. Journal of Infection and Public Health. 2014;**7**(4):323-332. DOI: 10.1016/j.jiph.2014.03.008

[35] Hudson JB. Applications of the phytomedicine *Echinacea purpurea* (Purple Coneflower) in infectious diseases. Journal of Biomedicine & Biotechnology. 2012;**2012**:769896. DOI: 10.1155/2012/769896

[36] Nabavi SM, Marchese A, Izadi M, Curti V, Daglia M, Nabavi SF. Plants belonging to the genus Thymus as antibacterial agents: From farm to pharmacy. Food Chemistry. 2015;**173**: 339-347. DOI: 10.1016/j.foodchem.2014.10.042

[37] Spînu M, Gurzău AE, Sandru CD, Gati G, Niculae M. Heavy metal pollutome and microbial resistome reciprocal interaction and its impact on human and animal matrices. In: Savić S, editor. Antibiotic Use in Animals. Rijeka, Croatia: InTech; 2018. pp. 135-154. DOI: 10.5772/intechopen.68438.ch8

[38] Tang SS, Prodhan ZH, Biswas SK, Le CF, Sekaran SD. Antimicrobial peptides from different plant sources: Isolation, characterisation, and purification. Phytochemistry. 2018;**154**: 94-105. DOI: 10.1016/j.phytochem.2018.07.002

[39] Nabavi SF, Di Lorenzo A, Izadi M, Sobarzo-Sánchez E, Daglia M, Nabavi SM. Antibacterial effects of cinnamon: From farm to food, cosmetic and pharmaceutical industries. Nutrients. 2015;**7**(9):7729-7748. DOI: 10.3390/nu7095359

[40] Mora A, Viso S, López C, Alonso MP, García-Garrote F, Dabhi G, et al. Poultry as reservoir for extraintestinal pathogenic *Escherichia coli* O45:K1:H7-B2-ST95 in humans. Veterinary Microbiology. 2013;**167**(3-4):506-512. DOI: 10.1016/j.vetmic.2013.08.007

[41] Benedec D, Oniga I, Hanganu D, Gheldiu AM, Pușcaș C, Silaghi-Dumitrescu R, et al. Sources for developing new medicinal products: Biochemical investigations on alcoholic extracts obtained from aerial parts of some Romanian Amaryllidaceae species. BMC Complementary and Alternative Medicine. 2018;**18**:226. DOI: 10.1186/s12906-018-2292-8

[42] Guh AY, Bulens SN, Mu Y, Jacob JT, Reno J, Scott J, et al. Epidemiology of carbapenem-resistant Enterobacteriaceae in 7 US communities, 2012–2013. Journal of the American Medical Association. 2015;**314**(14):1479-1487. DOI: 10.1001/jama.2015.12480

[43] Kotan R, Cakir A, Dadasoglu F, Aydin T, Cakmakci R, Ozer H, et al. Antibacterial activities of essential oils and extracts of Turkish Achillea, Satureja and Thymus species against plant pathogenic bacteria. Journal of the Science of Food and Agriculture. 2010;**90**(1):145-160. DOI: 10.1002/jsfa.3799

[44] Giacometti F, Magarotto J, Serraino A, Piva S. Highly suspected cases of salmonellosis in two cats fed with a commercial raw meat-based diet: Health risks to animals and zoonotic implications. BMC Veterinary Research. 2017;**13**(1):224. DOI: 10.1186/s12917-017-1143-z

[45] Voss-Rech D, Potter L, Silveira Luiz Vaz C, Brayer Pereira DI, Sangioni LA, Castagna Vargas A, et al. Antimicrobial resistance in nontyphoidal Salmonella isolated from human and poultry-related samples in Brazil: 20-year meta-analysis. Foodborne Pathogens and Disease. 2016;**20**(20):1-9. DOI: 10.1089/fpd.2016.2228

[46] Veeresham C. Natural products derived from plants as a source of drugs. Journal of Advanced Pharmaceutical Technology & Research. 2012;**3**(4):200-201. DOI: 10.4103/2231-4040.104709

[47] Integrated Surveillance of Antimicrobial Resistance in Foodborne Bacteria: Application of a One Health Approach. Geneva: World Health Organization; 2017. Licence: CC BY-NC-SA 3.0 IGO

[48] Braedel-Ruoff S. Immunomodulatory effects of *Viscum album* extracts on natural killer cells: Review of clinical trials. Forschende Komplementärmedizin. 2010;**17**(2):63-73. DOI: 10.1159/000288702

[49] Davin-Regli A, Pagès J-M. *Enterobacter aerogenes* and *Enterobacter cloacae*; versatile bacterial pathogens confronting antibiotic treatment. Frontiers in Microbiology;**6**:392. DOI: 10.3389/fmicb.2015.00392

[50] https://www.cdc.gov/onehealth/basics/zoonotic-diseases.html

[51] Leonard EK, Pearl DL, Finley RL, Janecko N, Peregrine AS, Reid-Smith RJ, et al. Evaluation of pet-related management factors and the risk of *Salmonella* spp. carriage in pet dogs from volunteer households in Ontario (2005–2006). Zoonoses and Public Health. 2011; **58**(2):140-149. DOI: 10.1111/j.1863-2378.2009.01320.x

[52] Poirel L, Kampfer P, Nordmann P. Chromosome-encoded Ambler class A beta-lactamase of *Kluyvera georgiana*, a probable progenitor of a subgroup of CTX-M extended spectrum β-lactamases. Antimicrobial Agents and Chemotherapy. 2002;**46**:4038-4040

[53] Luo Y, Cobb RE, Zhao H. Recent advances in natural product discovery. Current Opinion in Biotechnology. 2014 Dec;**30**:230-237. DOI: 10.1016/j.copbio.2014.09.002

[54] Liu Y, McKeever LC, Malik NS. Assessment of the antimicrobial activity of olive leaf extract against foodborne bacterial pathogens. Frontiers in Microbiology. 2017;**8**:113. DOI: 10.3389/fmicb.2017.00113

[55] Managing public health risks at the human-animal-environment interface [Internet]. 2018. Available from: http://www.who.int/zoonoses/en/ [Accessed: 2018-02-01]

[56] Goerge T, Lorenz MB, van Alen S, Hübner NO, Becker K, Köck R. MRSA colonization and infection among persons with occupational livestock exposure in Europe: Prevalence, preventive options and evidence. Veterinary Microbiology. 2017;**200**:6-12. DOI: 10.1016/j.vetmic.2015.10.027

[57] Liu Q, Meng X, Li Y, Zhao CN, Tang GY, Li HB. Antibacterial and antifungal activities of spices. International Journal of Molecular Sciences. 2017;**18**(6). DOI: 10.3390/ijms18061283

[58] Van Lochem S, Thompson PN, Annandale CH. Prevalence of methicillin-resistant *Staphylococcus aureus* among large commercial pig herds in South Africa. The Onderstepoort Journal of Veterinary Research. 2018;**85**(1):e1-e4. DOI: 10.4102/ojvr.v85i1.1561

[59] Guo A, He D, Xu HB, Geng CA, Zhao J. Promotion of regulatory T cell induction by immunomodulatory herbal medicine licorice and its two constituents. Scientific Reports. 2015;**5**:14046. DOI: 10.1038/srep14046

[60] Knapp CW, Mccluskey SM, Singh BK, Campbell CD, Hudson G, Graham DW. Antibiotic resistance gene abundances correlate with metal and geochemical conditions in archived Scottish soils. PLoS One. 2011;**6**:e27300. DOI: 10.1371/journal.pone.0027300

[61] Tomazi T, Coura FM, Gonçalves JL, Heinemann MB, Santos MV. Antimicrobial susceptibility patterns of *Escherichia coli* phylogenetic groups isolated from bovine clinical mastitis. Journal of Dairy Science. 2018. DOI: 10.3168/jds.2018-14485

[62] Antimicrobial Resistance: Global Report on Surveillance. France: WHO Library Cataloguing-in-Publication Data; 2014

[63] Gupta PD, Birdi TJ. Development of botanicals to combat antibiotic resistance. Journal of Ayurveda and Integrative Medicine. 2017;**8**(4):266-275. DOI: 10.1016/j.jaim.2017.05.004

[64] Falsafi T, Moradi P, Mahboubi M, Rahimi E, Momtaz H, Hamedi B. Chemical composition and anti-*Helicobacter pylori* effect of *Satureja bachtiarica* Bunge essential oil. Phytomedicine. 2015;**22**(1):173-177. DOI: 10.1016/j.phymed.2014.11.012

[65] Hille K, Möbius N, Akmatov MK, Verspohl J, Rabold D, Hartmann M, et al. Zoonoses research in the German National Cohort: Feasibility of parallel sampling of pets and

owners. Bundesgesundheitsblatt, Gesundheitsforschung, Gesundheitsschutz. 2014;**57**(11): 1277-1282. DOI: 10.1007/s00103-014-2047-8

[66] van Bree FPJ, Bokken GCAM, Mineur R, Franssen F, Opsteegh M, van der Giessen JWB, et al. Zoonotic bacteria and parasites found in raw meat-based diets for cats and dogs. The Veterinary Record. 2018;**182**(2):50. DOI: 10.1136/vr.104535

[67] Radji M, Agustama RA, Elya B, Tjampakasari CR. Antimicrobial activity of green tea extract against isolates of methicillin-resistant *Staphylococcus aureus* and multi-drug resistant *Pseudomonas aeruginosa*. Asian Pacific Journal of Tropical Biomedicine. 2013;**3**(8):663-667; discussion 666. DOI: 10.1016/S2221-1691(13)60133-1

[68] Feltrin F, Alba P, Kraushaar B, Ianzano A, Argudín MA, Di Matteo P, et al. A livestock-associated, multidrug-resistant, methicillin-resistant *Staphylococcus aureus* clonal complex 97 lineage spreading in dairy cattle and pigs in Italy. Applied and Environmental Microbiology. 2015;**82**(3):816-821. DOI: 10.1128/AEM.02854-15

[69] Wang M, Zhao S, Zhu P, Nie C, Ma S, Wang N, et al. Purification, characterization and immunomodulatory activity of water extractable polysaccharides from the swollen culms of *Zizania latifolia*. International Journal of Biological Macromolecules. 2018;**107**(Pt A):882-890. DOI: 10.1016/j.ijbiomac.2017.09.062

[70] Dall'Acqua S, Perissutti B, Grabnar I, Farra R, Comar M, Agostinis C, et al. Pharmacokinetics and immunomodulatory effect of lipophilic Echinacea extract formulated in softgel capsules. European Journal of Pharmaceutics and Biopharmaceutics. 2015;**97**(Pt A):8-14. DOI: 10.1016/j.ejpb.2015.09.021

[71] Walsh F. Investigating antibiotic resistance in non-clinical environments. Frontiers in Microbiology. 2013;**4**:19. DOI: 10.3389/fmicb.2013.00019

[72] Kruse H, kirkemo AM, Handeland K. Wildlife as source of zoonotic infections. Emerging Infectious Diseases. 2004;**10**(12):2067-2072. Review

[73] Becker K, Ballhausen B, Kahl BC, Köck R. The clinical impact of livestock-associated methicillin-resistant *Staphylococcus aureus* of the clonal complex 398 for humans. Veterinary Microbiology. 2017;**200**:33-38. DOI: 10.1016/j.vetmic.2015.11.013

[74] Brennan GI, Abbott Y, Burns A, Leonard F, McManus BA, O'Connell B, et al. The emergence and spread of multiple livestock-associated clonal complex 398 methicillin-resistant and methicillin-susceptible *Staphylococcus aureus* strains among animals and humans in the Republic of Ireland, 2010–2014. PLoS One. 2016;**11**(2):e0149396. DOI: 10.1371/journal.pone.0149396

[75] da Silva Menezes Azola J, de Souza Moreira B, da Silva Menezes F, Soares Horta de Souza C, Santos LA, Alves Rufino LR, et al. The antimicrobial activity of plant extract against *Staphylococcus aureus* isolated from cows milk samples with subclinical mastitis in Brazil. Journal of Agriculture and Veterinary Science. 2016;**9-10**:26-29

[76] Morwal S, Sharma SK. Bacterial Zoonosis. A Public Health Importance. Journal of Dairy, Veterinary & Animal Research. 2017;**5**(2):00135. DOI: 10.15406/jdvar.2017.05.00135

[77] Chen Q, Liu Z, He JH. *Achyranthes bidentata* polysaccharide enhances immune response in weaned piglets. Immunopharmacology and Immunotoxicology. 2009;**31**(2):253-260. DOI: 10.1080/08923970802439795

[78] Dapas B, Dall'Acqua S, Bulla R, Agostinis C, Perissutti B, Invernizzi S, et al. Immunomodulation mediated by a herbal syrup containing a standardized Echinacea root extract: A pilot study in healthy human subjects on cytokine gene expression. Phytomedicine. 2014; **21**(11):1406-1410. DOI: 10.1016/j.phymed.2014.04.034

[79] Donati V, Feltrin F, Hendriksen RS, Svendsen CA, Cordaro G, García-Fernández A, et al. Extended-spectrum-beta-lactamases, AmpC beta-lactamases and plasmid mediated quinolone resistance in *Klebsiella* spp. from companion animals in Italy. PLoS One. 2014;**9**(3): e90564. DOI: 10.1371/journal.pone.0090564

[80] Hagiwara S, Mori K, Okada H, Oikawa S, Nagahata H. Acute *Escherichia coli* mastitis in dairy cattle: Diagnostic parameters associated with poor prognosis. The Journal of Veterinary Medical Science. 2014;**76**(11):1431-1436. DOI: 10.1292/jvms.13-0610

[81] Tarr GAM, Shringi S, Oltean HN, Mayer J, Rabinowitz P, Wakefield J, et al. Importance of case age in the purported association between phylogenetics and hemolytic uremic syndrome in *Escherichia coli* O157:H7 infections. Epidemiology and Infection. 2018;**19**:1-6. DOI: 10.1017/S0950268818001632

[82] Wikaningtyas P, Sukandar EY. The antibacterial activity of selected plants towards resistant bacteria isolated from clinical specimens. Asian Pacific Journal of Tropical Biomedicine. 2016;**6**(1):16-19. DOI: 10.1016/j.apjtb.2015.08.003

[83] Köck R, Schaumburg F, Mellmann A, Köksal M, Jurke A, Becker K, et al. Livestock-associated methicillin-resistant *Staphylococcus aureus* (MRSA) as causes of human infection and colonization in Germany. PLoS One. 2013;**8**(2):e55040. DOI: 10.1371/journal.pone.0055040

[84] Niculae M, Spînu M, Şandru CD, Brudaşcã F, Cadar D, Szakacs B, et al. Antimicrobial potential of some Lamiaceae essential oils against animal multiresistant bacteria. Lucrari Stiintifice - Universitatea de Stiinte Agricole a Banatului Timisoara. Medicina Veterinara. 2009;**42**(1):170-175

[85] Baker-Austin C, Wright MS, Stepanauskas R, McArthur JV. Co-selection of antibiotic and metal resistance. Trends in Microbiology. 2006;**14**(4):176-182. DOI: 10.1016/j.tim.2006.02.006

[86] Damborg P, Broens EM, Chomel BB, Guenther S, Pasmans F, Wagenaar JA, et al. Bacterial zoonoses transmitted by household pets: State-of-the-art and future perspectives for targeted research and policy actions. Journal of Comparative Pathology. 2016;**155**(Suppl 1): S27-S40. DOI: 10.1016/j.jcpa.2015. 03.004

[87] Shin B, Park W. Zoonotic diseases and phytochemical medicines for microbial infections in veterinary science: Current state and future perspective. Frontiers in Veterinary Science. 2018;**5**:166. DOI: 10.3389/fvets.2018.00166

[88] Podder MP, Rogers L, Daley PK, Keefe GP, Whitney HG, Tahlan K. *Klebsiella* species associated with bovine mastitis in Newfoundland. PLoS One. 2014;**9**(9):e106518. DOI: 10.1371/journal.pone.0106518

[89] Novais A, Cantón R, Coque TM, Moya A, Baquero F, Galán JC. Mutational events in cefotaximase extended-spectrum beta-lactamases of the CTX-M-1 cluster involved in ceftazidime resistance. Antimicrobial Agents and Chemotherapy. 2008;**52**:2377-2382

[90] Peñalver P, Huerta B, Borge C, Astorga R, Romero R, Perea A. Antimicrobial activity of five essential oils against origin strains of the Enterobacteriaceae family. APMIS. 2005;**113**(1):1-6

[91] Amber R, Adnan M, Tariq A, Khan SN, Mussarat S, Hashem A, et al. Antibacterial activity of selected medicinal plants of northwest Pakistan traditionally used against mastitis in livestock. Saudi Journal of Biological Sciences. 2018;**25**(1):154-161. DOI: 10.1016/j.sjbs.2017.02.008

[92] Khan UA, Rahman H, Qasim M, Hussain A, Azizllah A, Murad W, et al. *Alkanna tinctoria* leaves extracts: A prospective remedy against multidrug resistant human pathogenic bacteria. BMC Complementary and Alternative Medicine. 2015;**15**:127. DOI: 10.1186/s12906-015-0646-z

[93] Giupana R, Niculae M, Pall E, Negruțiu V, Silvana P, Vasiu A, Pușcașu R, Șandru CD, Spînu M. Solvent nature influences the effects of *Melissa officinalis* extract on the milk microbiome in cows with subclinical mastitis, accepted for publication in Annals of Phytomedicine, December issue

Chapter 7

# Beneficial Microbes: Roles in the Era of Antimicrobial Resistance

Ayorinde O. Afolayan, Adewale Adetoye and
Funmilola A. Ayeni

Additional information is available at the end of the chapter

http://dx.doi.org/10.5772/intechopen.79635

**Abstract**

The upsurge of resistance in classes of antibiotics in varied bacterial species has increased the search for alternatives to antibiotics in bacterial infections. However, one alternative is the beneficial bacteria in foods, environment and gut. Probiotics is now being embraced as an alternative strategy to combat antibiotic resistant pathogens. A newer application is gut microbiota in its healthy state combating pathogenic and antibiotic resistant microbes. There have been numerous applications of beneficial bacteria against different infectious agents. This article describes the concept of beneficial microbes as antimicrobial agents with current applications as antimicrobial agents, various applications in the human gut with future directions.

**Keywords:** probiotics, lactic acid bacteria, alternative therapy, pathogens, applications

## 1. Introduction

Microorganisms exist from where we can imagine to places we least expect e.g. outer space and the dead sea. Much of the global atmospheric oxygen is as a result of microbial activity [1]. They also maintain the gut health by regulating the microflora, stimulating the development of the immune system, production and enhancement of some important nutrients [2] and there seem to be a natural interdependence of life on microorganisms.

At the time of antibiotic discovery, Fleming looked into the future and foresaw that antimicrobial resistance would be a challenge, and he gave a subtle warning about the potential impact of sub-optimal dosage in fostering antimicrobial resistance during his Nobel laureate acceptance speech. Unfortunately, about 10 years after Penicillin was discovered, Fleming's fears were confirmed when penicillin-resistant pathogens emerged. Since then (and for more than half of a century later), the discovery of a novel antibiotic has always been accompanied by the eventual emergence of antibiotic-resistant strains due to regular and inappropriate usage of antibiotics by humans [3]. Antimicrobial drug resistance is a global threat to public health and human activities contribute significantly to the selection of resistant strains through non prudent use of these antimicrobial agents giving rise to the development of a generation of antimicrobial resistant mutants circulating in the biosphere [3]. Unfortunately, resistance has eventually been seen to nearly all antibiotics that have been developed [4].

## 2. Probiotics

"Probiotics are live microorganisms which when administered in adequate amount confer a health benefit on the host" [5]. The concept of probiotics evolved from the work of Elie Metchnikoff in the early twentieth century when he observed that certain beneficial microbes particularly lactic acid bacteria in milk consumed by peasant Bulgarians were responsible for their longevity. Lactic acid bacteria and Bifidobacteria are the most commonly used organisms as probiotics, although some other bacteria such as *Escherichia coli* Nissle 1917 [6] and yeast such as *Saccharomyces boulardii* are also used [7]. *Lactobacillus* spp. being an integral part of the intestinal microflora having earned the "Generally Regarded as Safe" status are the most successful probiotic candidates. Lactic acid producing bacteria are known to possess various health benefits such as anti-cancer activity, lowering of serum cholesterol, lactose intolerance alleviation, prevention of antibiotic related diarrhea, stimulation of the immune functions, antimicrobial activity against resistant pathogens [8, 9] prevention and treatment of Inflammatory bowel disease [10], respiratory viral infection [11]. Recently, *Lactobacillus* spp. have also been reported to have beneficial effects in patients suffering psychological disorders, such as depression and anxiety [12–14]. Probiotics have been proposed to exert health benefits through several mechanisms [15], these include enhancement of the epithelial barrier, increased adhesion to intestinal mucosa, and concomitant inhibition of pathogen adhesion, competitive exclusion of pathogenic microorganisms, production of antimicrobial substances and modulation of the immune system. For example, *E. coli* Nissle 1917 has been used as an alternative treatment option of Ulcerative colitis—a chronic intestinal disease [16]. Generally, LAB and probiotics augment the antagonistic activity of the gut commensals against infectious agents, including the opportunistic pathogen *Clostridium difficile* that is implicated in antibiotic-associated diarrhea [17]. Other probiotics have been confirmed to prevent intestinal infections (such as stomach infections caused by *Helicobacter pylori*) and extra-intestinal infections (such as infections of the respiratory tract). This way, the spread of antibiotic resistance diminishes drastically, and the gut microbiota structure and overall health of the host is restored. This bodes well for the future of the human race. The probiotic properties are strain specific and cannot be extrapolated to other strains of the same species, also the organisms are to be administered live hence, they must be safe and produce the desired beneficial effect [18]. There are critical guidelines on the minimum requirement for the selection of probiotic strains as recommended by Food and Agricultural Organization of the World Health Organization [5] and can be summarized as;

### 2.1. Identification of genus, species and strain

Since the probiotic property is a strain specific attribute, it will be important to link specific health benefit to a particular strain and also for epidemiological surveillance purposes, the proposed microorganism must be identified to the strain level, the strains should be correctly identified using both phenotypic and genotypic methods and deposited in an internationally recognized culture collection [19], molecular methods such as DNA/DNA hybridization and 16S rRNA gene sequencing are suggested for strain identification.

### 2.2. Assessment of safety

Selected strain must be non-pathogenic, non-haemolytic and non-toxic in the intended host. They must be safe and qualify for the qualified presumption of safety (QPS) as stipulated by European Food Safety Authority. The antibiotic resistance susceptibility pattern including the MIC to antibiotics of medical importance should be determined, the intended strain should not possess antimicrobial resistance determinants [18]. Probiotic strains should also be assessed for metabolic activities such as production of D-lactate and bile salt deconjugation. Assessment of toxin production should be done for microbial strains that belong to species that are known to produce mammalian toxins. The demonstration of lack of infectivity of the probiotic strain in animals with deficient immune functions will further substantiate the safety profile of such strain. A post market epidemiological surveillance of adverse effects in the host is also an important safety requirement.

### 2.3. Functional considerations

#### *2.3.1. Resistance to bile salt and gastric conditions*

Probiotic strains intended for oral administration must be able to survive passage through the gastrointestinal tract of the host, where they will encounter an hostile condition characterized with low pH and bile salt and must survive in adequate amount to confer health benefit on the host. Lactic acid bacteria isolated from the guts tends to better survive this route than those isolated from other sources [9].

#### *2.3.2. Ability to adhere and colonize the epithelial cells and tissues*

The ability of the probiotic strain to adhere to intestinal mucosa and epithelial cells is an important characteristic for its colonization and survival in the host. Successful colonization of the intestinal mucosa by probiotics is important for immune modulation and inhibition of pathogens by competitive exclusion. Microorganisms that have poor adherence to epithelial cells will easily be washed away and unlikely to colonize the host for a probiotic effect [9].

#### *2.3.3. In vivo validation of health benefits*

Probiotics must be able to exert health benefits through their activities in the host, in vitro tests to predict the health benefits to host may not be sufficient. *In vivo* experiments should be carried out to validate *in vitro* health benefit potentials.

### 2.4. Overview of approved probiotic strains currently used

Health agencies in different countries have specific microorganisms approved as probiotics. For example, Health Canada approves the use of *Lactobacillus johnsonii* La1, Lj1, or NCC 533 strains (to treat *Helicobacter pylori* infections), *Lactobacillus rhamnosus* GG (for prevention/management of antibiotic-associated diarrhea), and *Saccharomyces boulardii/S. cerevisiae* (for prevention/management of antibiotic-associated diarrhea) in doses of $\geq 10^7$ colony forming units (CFU) daily [20]. Other probiotics strains has also been approved by Health Canada [20]. US FDA also have a comprehensive list of approved probiotic metabolites for use as food ingredients or additives after they have been certified as GRAS e.g. *Streptomyces natalensis* and *Streptomyces chattanoogensis* in Natamycin [21]. A probiotic strain is usually identified with internationally approved methods; by the genus, species, subspecies (where applicable), and the specific strain designated with an alphanumeric identity e.g. *Lactobacillus casei* DN-114. Probiotic strain designation is vital, since health benefit(s) to the host must be linked to the particular strain or a combination of strains and these benefits are strain specific. The WHO/FAO guideline stipulates that probiotic strains should be registered in an internationally recognized culture collection [5].

*Lactobacillus* and Bifidobacteria species are the most commonly used probiotic microorganisms, however, some strains of *Escherichia coli*, Bacillus species and the yeast *Saccharomyces boulardii* are also used. Recently, *Clostridium butyricum* was also approved for probiotic use in European Union [22].

### 2.5. Challenges encountered in formulation and use of probiotics

Due to the well-known benefits of probiotics, food companies incorporate probiotics into foods (termed functional foods) for greater marketability [23]. However, there is always a tendency for these probiotic strains to be lost or greatly reduced in number and viability during food processing and/or storage such that the purported health benefit is eventually lost. Thus, probiotic instability is one challenge faced by food formulators and manufacturers that intend to incorporate probiotic strains into their product. The shelf life is mostly unpredictable, so much that excess of up to 200% viable cells are added in probiotic products to make-up for cells that die before it reaches the consumer, this makes backing up label claims difficult and also increases the production cost. Manufacturers also have to prove that the probiotics will still remain stable and viable within the human body in adequate amounts until they reach the gut where their impact is the greatest [23].

### 2.6. Antimicrobial activities against pathogens

The ability of the proposed probiotic strain to produce antimicrobial substances against pathogens is an important consideration in the selection of probiotic strains. Lactic acid bacteria produce antimicrobial metabolic compounds during lactic fermentation such as hydrogen peroxides, organic acids such as lactic, acetic and propionic acid. Bacteriocins and other proteinaceous inhibitory substances are also produced by some probiotic organisms [24].

#### 2.6.1. *Organic acids*

The end product of fermentation of lactic acid bacteria include organic acids such as lactic acid, acetic acid, propionic acid, butyric acid etc. which reduces the pH of their growth medium and thus makes it unfavorable for the growth of other competing microorganisms. The organic acids exert their antimicrobial activity by interfering with the integrity of the cell membrane, inhibition of various metabolic functions and active transport, lowering of intracellular pH [25].

#### 2.6.2. *Hydrogen peroxide*

Lactic acid bacteria do not utilize the cytochrome system as a result of lack of the heme group and thus cannot reduce oxygen to water leading to the production of hydrogen peroxide from the action of flavoprotein oxidases or NAD peroxides. The hydrogen peroxide is produced in amount capable of bacterial antagonism particularly against species which lack catalase peroxidase. Free radicals such as hydroxyl radical and superoxides which can damage bacteria DNA may also have hydrogen peroxide as precursor for their production. Lactic acid bacteria had been reported to produce hydrogen peroxide as part of its inhibitory mechanisms [9].

#### 2.6.3. *Bacteriocin*

Some lactic acid bacteria produce small, heat-stable, ribosomally synthesized inhibitory bioactive peptides produced during their primary phase of growth called bacteriocin. Many bacteriocins exhibit a narrow spectrum of antimicrobial activity, particularly against bacteria strains of species related to the bacteriocin producing species while some display activity across a variety of different bacteria genera. Bacteriocins exhibit a wide diversity as regards their structure, size, mechanism of action, inhibitory spectrum and target cell receptors [26]. Most of the bacteriocins produced by LAB appears to have a narrow spectrum of antimicrobial activity, however nisin and pediocin are known to exhibit a broad antibacterial spectrum [23]. Bacteriocins are easily degraded by proteolytic enzymes particularly by those produced by the guts of mammals which make them safe for human use [27]. Generally, bacteriocins can be sub-divided into three classes according to their structure and mode of antibacterial action. Class I bacteriocins include nisin, which is active against Gram positive bacteria including food spoilage and pathogenic microbes. Nisin has a pentacyclic structure composed of 34 amino acids with one lanthionine residue (Ring A) and four beta-methyllanthionine residues (rings B, C, D, E), heat stable at 121°C but becomes less heat stable on prolong heating, especially between pH 5 and 7 [27]. Bacteriocin has proven to be an efficient natural antimicrobial agent against pathogens and food spoilage bacteria, including *Listeria monocytogenes, Staphylococcus aureus, Bacillus cereus* and *Clostridium botulinum* [28].

Enterocin X, plantaricin A and lactococcin G are class 2b bacteriocins commonly produced by *Enterococcus faecium* and lysostaphin, enterolysin A, helveticin J are common class 3 bacteriocins produced by *Lactobacillus helveticus,* they are heat stable with a large molecular weight of more than 30 kDa [29]. Nisin is the only bacteriocin that has been officially approved for use in the food industry [30], class II bacteriocins are relatively small, heat-stable and contain peptides while Class III bacteriocins are heat stable and also have a relatively large molecular weight [27]. The classes of bacteriocins produced by Gram-positive beneficial bacteria include lantibiotics and non-lantibiotic heat stable proteins [31] while Gram-negative bacteria produce colicin and microcin [32].

### *2.6.4. Prebiotics*

Prebiotics are non-digestible food products that increase the relative abundance of beneficial microorganisms in the gut when ingested. Similar to the influence of complex plant polysaccharides on the gut microbiota composition and beneficial metabolite production, prebiotics enhance the production of short chain fatty acids such as butyrate—a metabolite that serves as an energy source for colonic epithelium. Examples of prebiotics used include inulin, fructooligosaccharides, and galactooligosaccharides, Some of these prebiotics are found naturally in foods (such as barley, wheat), and in garlic and raw onions. These prebiotics have been applied in malnourished Thai children and children from certain countries in Africa [33], South America and Europe in order to improve the adsorption of calcium as well as improvement of growth [34].

## 3. Synbiotics

Synbiotics is a term used for the combined use of probiotics and prebiotics to achieve a more efficient impact on the gut microbiota [34]. This concept surfaced in order to tackle possible difficulty of the probiotics to establish itself in the gut. In this case, prebiotics and probiotics are co-administered in order to improve the growth/relative abundance and establishment of probiotics in the gastrointestinal tract of its host. The probiotic strains used in conjunction with prebiotics include Lactobacilli and Bifidobacilli, while the prebiotics used along with probiotic strains include inulin, galactooligosaccharide, and fructooligosaccharide. The combination of probiotics and prebiotics in therapy helps to give stability to the gut microbiota, which translates to overall health of the host's gut and the host in general. This combination also helps to enhance antimicrobial activity, and the combined effect includes; competition with the pathogen for adherence sites, production of metabolites that are toxic to the pathogens, production of compounds that degrade toxins produced by the pathogens, obstruction of attachment sites and toxin receptors, and modulation of the immune system to respond effectively to pathogen invasion [35].

## 4. Antimicrobial potentials of beneficial microbes against antibiotic resistant strains

The antimicrobial activities of beneficial microorganisms particularly lactic acid bacteria isolated from various sources against pathogens have been reported by many authors [7, 36].

Afolayan et al. [37] isolated lactic acid bacteria from different variety of "*Ogi*" a fermented cereal in western part of Nigeria with antimicrobial activities against various gastrointestinal pathogens. *Shigella* spp. are enteric pathogens which cause dysentery and diarrhea and are a leading cause of gastroenteritis- associated deaths in about 3–5 million under 5 years old children in developing countries [38, 39]. Lactic acid bacteria strongly inhibited gastrointestinal *E. coli* in co culture [40]. Cell free supernatant of *Lactobacillus casei* isolated from traditional yoghurt and milk was reported to strongly inhibit multi-drug resistant *Shigella sonnei* and *S. flexneri* [39], and also starter cultures in Nigerian yoghurt and the yoghurt itself has been reported to have strong inhibitory effects on gastrointestinal pathogens [41]. Salmonellosis contributes significantly to global morbidity and mortality. There are about 93.4 million cases of salmonellosis worldwide resulting in 155,000 death annually [42], *Lactobacillus* spp. with antimicrobial activity against *Salmonella typhi* were isolated by Abdel-Daim et al. [43] and *in vivo* anti-salmonella activities of lactobacilli has also been reported by Casey et al. [44] in pigs. Antimicrobial activities of lactic acid bacteria has also been reported against *Pseudomonas aeruginosa, Providencia vermicola, Alcaligenes faecalis* and MRSA in co culture [45].

The increasing emergence of antibiotic resistant uropathogens, yeast infection and recurrent infection has necessitated special interest in the antibacterial activity of lactic acid bacteria against uropathogens [46]. There are increasing scientific evidences that LAB can prevent the growth and attachment of pathogens to epithelial cells [47]. It was reported by Adeniyi et al. [48] that lactic acid bacteria isolated from various Nigerian based fermented foods exhibited varying antimicrobial activity against organisms implicated in urinary tract infections. *Weissella* spp. isolated from African fermented food and cow intestine demonstrated significant inhibitory activity against multi drug resistant uropathogens [7]. Lactic acid bacteria isolated from a menstruating Nigerian woman was shown to have antimicrobial activity against an array of uropathogens; *Escherichia coli, Proteus mirabilis* 42P, *Pseudomonas aeruginosa, Citrobacter freundii* and *Enterobacter cloacae* [49]. The organic acid produced by lactic acid bacteria has been proven to be inhibitory to *Neisseria gonorrhoeae* [50]. The antibacterial activity of lactic acid bacteria isolated from selected Nigerian vegetables against *Pseudomonas aeruginosa, Escherichia coli, Proteus penneri,* and *Enterococcus faecalis* was published by Bamidele et al. [51]. *Lactobacillus* spp. have been reported to inhibit the growth of *Candida albicans* and prevent the relapse of yeast infection [52]. The metabolite of *Lactobacillus plantarum* strain N4 was discovered to possess antiviral activities against coronavirus causing gastroenteritis [53], certain lactic acid bacteria have been suggested to be effective in reducing the severity and duration of acute rotavirus gastroenteritis [54].

## 5. Beneficial microbes in the gut; effects on antibiotic resistant strains

In the gut lies a community of beneficial microorganisms that have carved a niche and have evolved with humans over several generations—collectively known as the gut microbiota. Microorganisms that make up the gut microbiota include members of bacteria, fungi, viruses, archaea, and protists. Before the advent of next-generation sequencing technologies, very little was known about the composition and functions of this microbial community, and as such were not thought as agents to be considered in health and disease. Now, we are just beginning to scratch the surface of the potentials of this novel 'organ', and its implication in the overall health of humans. It is referred to as an 'organ' because the gut microbiome (the gut microbiota, gut microbial genomes, and the living environment) is made of millions of bacterial cells that collectively weigh about 1.5 kg, possesses about 150 times more genes than human genes, and contribute significantly to human health. As a result of advances in research, scientists are beginning to appreciate the beneficial roles of gut microbes, and their symbiotic relationship with us, their host. Although previously thought to be responsible for the production of essential vitamins B and K alone, the gut microbiota has been discovered to be implicated in various aspect of human health, and its effects extend beyond the gastrointestinal tract through the release of biosynthesized metabolites (by the gut microbes) from the gut into the systemic circulation. For example, the response of immune cells to inflammation is modulated by the gut microbiota [55]. The effect of these metabolites extends even to the central nervous system where they influence behavior, mood, and emotions.

In the gastrointestinal tract, the gut microbiota protects the gut against invading pathogens by competing with them for nutrients and attachment site. Most of the antibiotic-resistant disease-causing infectious agents that invade the gastrointestinal tract are food-borne or water-borne, and they include *Salmonella, Shigella, Campylobacter,* and *Listeria monocytogenes*. On the other hand, the gut microbiota is dominated by members of the Firmicutes, Bacteroidetes, Proteobacteria, and Actinobacteria. Other less dominant bacterial phyla include the Fusobacteria, Tenericutes, Spirochaetes (differentially abundant in the gut of hunter-gatherers and rural individuals who consume plant-based foods), Elusimicrobia, and Verrucomicrobia. *Prevotella*—a member of the phylum Bacteroidetes—has also been found to be more abundant in individuals whose lifestyle resembles those of the Paleolithic (such as the hunter-gatherers) and Neolithic (such as the subsistence agriculturalists) era. Conversely, *Bacteroides*—another member of Bacteroidetes—is more abundant in populations that practice a westernized lifestyle, characterized by high-fat, low-fiber diet. Many of the gut commensals such as *Eubacterium, Ruminococcus, Roseburia,* and *Faecalibacterium* are members of the Firmicutes that produce short-chain fatty acids (such as butyrate, acetate, and propionate) as a product of microbial fermentation (the breakdown of complex polysaccharides), and these acids diminish diarrhea and gastrointestinal inflammation. These short chain fatty acids (SCFA) also create a harsh environment for the colonization of invading gastrointestinal pathogens by the reduction of intestinal pH. Other pathogen-inhibiting metabolites produced by gut commensals include phenols, ammonia, bacteriocins, and ammonia [56].

The composition of the gut microbiota can be positively or negatively affected by dietary habits and other lifestyle factors, the use of antibiotics, age, the state of health, and surgery amongst other factors [57]. The regular consumption of a fiber-rich, plant-based diet improves the compositional profile of the gut microbiota in terms of richness and diversity, and also improves the functional capabilities of the members of the gut microbiota. Good lifestyle practices such as the consumption of fiber-rich foods and fruits increases the relative abundance of beneficial gut microbes which produce metabolites that are responsible for overall gut epithelial health [58]. The impact of diet on the stability of the gut microbiota cannot be overemphasized. This is because an imbalance in the structure of the gut microbiota is a risky phenomenon in the development of gastrointestinal and extra-gastrointestinal diseases. Antibiotics do not differentiate between beneficial bacteria and pathogenic bacteria, and as such, there is a significant decrease in the richness and diversity of the gut microbiota after antibiotic administration. This places a fatal dent on gut microbiota stability and creates an environment for opportunistic pathogens such as antibiotic-associated *Clostridium difficile* to thrive resulting in diarrhea. Dysbiosis (impairment in the natural balance) of the gut microbiota has been associated not only with the risk of antibiotic-associated diarrhea, but a plethora of other diseases such as type 2 diabetes, cancer, obesity, inflammatory bowel diseases and irritable bowel syndrome [59]. Adulthood is generally characterized by a stable gut microbiota, with occasional shifts in gut microbial diversity due to change in dietary habits, medication, illness or travel. On the other hand, the gut microbiota of infants is quite volatile and changes rapidly depending on the mode of birth, whether they are breast-fed or formula-fed, and whether they have been weaned or not. By the age of 2–5 years, their gut microbiota begins to resemble that of a typical adult. At the tail end of life, age-related changes in physiology of the body and changes in dietary habits due to loss of dentition could have a negative impact on the gut microbiota thereby making it less stable [60]. At this age also, the use of medication is high because they are more prone to diseases and impairments, which could influence gut microbial profiles. All of these factors mentioned above have to be considered when designing strategies aimed at restoring or contributing to the natural balance of the gut microbiota.

## 6. Current applications

The beneficial role played by bacteria in ingested fermented foods was linked to increased longevity in Balkans [61]. The administration of probiotics has also reduced the shedding of a pathogenic serotype of *E. coli* (*E. coli* O157: H7) by farm animals, thereby reducing the spread of these resistant strains from animals to humans who handle them regularly [62]. Also, there is hope that probiotics wills soon replace antibiotics in the veterinary field to treat diseases of farm animals while enhancing the growth of these farm animals. This way, antibiotic-resistant zoonotic pathogens do not re-emerge and enter the food chain. Also, the cost of production and maintenance of livestock will drop significantly if probiotics are being utilized rather than antibiotics.

Researchers and clinicians are getting conscious of the fact that probiotics isolated from the host have a higher tendency to remain endogenous when administered than probiotics gotten from other sources. This fact informs their decision on the choice of probiotics to be administered. Capsules of probiotics are sometimes used in concert with antibiotics to treat particular diseases with greater effect than if either of them (probiotics or antibiotics) was used alone [17]. This co-administration is done with the hope that this action will reduce antibiotic selective pressure, and decrease the emergence of drug-resistant pathogens. Currently, research is ongoing on the packaging of lyophilized lactic acid bacteria into capsules so that they can be used in the veterinary field (as probiotics) to inhibit the proliferation of zoonotic pathogens [36]. This method will limit the spread of diseases from animals to humans through animal-derived products. Probiotics have been introduced into milk, formula, and other infant foods as a supplement, in order to improve the human gut microbiota stability and tap into the purported benefits of probiotics. The viability of probiotics is enhanced in its lyophilized state within low-fat milk or fruit juice by food formulators and manufacturers [22]. The improvement of the viability of probiotic strains can also be achieved by microcapsulation—a formulation approach that employs the use of microcapsules to package solids, liquids, or gases where these contents could be released in a controlled manner under specific conditions [22]. With this technique, the formulation, storage, and successful transport of probiotic strains to their destination in the gut is assured. Although probiotics are generally regarded as safe, there is a conscious effort to confirm that they do not carry and transfer genes conferring antimicrobial resistance, as this will defeat the purpose of probiotics usage [63]. By and large, the ultimate aim of the use of probiotics is to ensure the stability of the human and animal gut microbiota so as to take advantage of the symbiotic activity of the probiotic and the gut microbial community in the fight against multi-drug resistant gastrointestinal pathogens [8].

Probiotics are most commonly sold as foods or food supplements, powders, lozenges, tablets (could be chewable, enterocoated or not), sticks, capsules, bottle caps, sachets, stick packs, and oil suspensions (usually for babies) probiotic nasal spray and ointments have also been developed. Most probiotic products available in the market are dairy based foods, including fermented milks, yogurts, cheese etc. The health claims on most probiotics labels tend to be general and such products are intended for the general healthy population. However, manufacturers, food companies, and the media have dispersed unproven information about the purported health benefits of probiotics even before a comprehensive clinical trial has been conducted to validate the efficacy, and the risk–benefit association In terms of probiotics acceptability, although probiotics have been used in the food industries for decades, the discovery of novel strains and genetic manipulation of known strains (some of which are pathogenic) is usually accompanied with a mirror image of the consumer skepticism associated with the marketing of genetically modified foods.

Another current application of beneficial gut microbes is the method of fecal microbiota transplantation (FMT). Fecal microbiota transplantation is a technique that involves the reconstitution of the deliberately-emptied gut of gastrointestinal-diseased patients with the gut microbiota of healthy donor as a therapeutic alternative measure to antibiotic administration for the restoration of the healthy gut microbiota [64]. This method has enabled the majority of those who have been suffering from antibiotic-associated diarrhea and inflammatory bowel diseases to lead a normal life after treatment. Although the filtered donor stool suspension can be passed into the gut of the recipient through rectal enema, nasoduodenal tube, or the nasogastric tube, colonoscopy is the most preferred method of stool suspension transfer. These donor stools could also be lyophilized and packaged into capsules, to be used in treating gastrointestinal infections. Stool banks are currently available in Europe and North America for the storage of tested, pathogen-free donor stools until they are needed by the medical practitioners [65]. Knowledge about the microbial composition of each donor stool and other components of the stool will also inform the medical practitioner and the patient on what to expect after transplantation. Due to the fact that the mental receptiveness of the fecal microbiota transplantation by the patient could have an effect on the effectiveness of this procedure, and the fact that there is a risk of undetected pathogens/diseases transfer from the donor to the recipient, some scientists advocate for an alternative to FMT. They believe that isolation and identification of the key players in the restoration of gut microbiota balance will help in the design of a consortium of these microbial players. An artificial stool could be prepared using this donor-sourced purified consortium of gut bacteria which would then replace the use of the donor stools in a less risky, more efficient and more mentally-acceptable manner [66]. This burgeoning field is known as Microbial Ecosystem Therapeutics.

## 7. Future directions

As previously mentioned, MET is one proposed alternative to FMT. Apart from the fact that this procedure is less disgusting and less risky than FMT, it has the potential to be regulated and standardized more efficiently than FMT [67]. MET procedure involves the isolation, characterization, and screening of gut microbes (for antibiotic resistance, presence of virulence determinants, etc.) from a healthy donor. Gut microbes that pass the screening test will then be recombined into a microbial ecosystem where their combined efforts and synergistic relationships will be more effective in tackling invasive enteropathogens and opportunistic pathogens such as *Clostridium difficile* [68]. In the future, this consortium of synergistic gut microorganisms will be packaged and lyophilized in their live form into capsules and prescribed as a drug. MET is still in its infancy, and it also has to go through regulatory procedures just like a drug, and standardized before it is globally accepted for use in treating gastrointestinal diseases such as antibiotic-induced diarrhea as a therapeutic alternative measure to antibiotic administration. Nevertheless, it offers a promising and a more effective alternative to the use of FMT. Furthermore, since the exact composition of the consortium is defined, it will be easy to track the long-term effect of this potential drug on human health. Also, questions about the interaction between the consortium and the resident gut microbiota and their combined effect on the health of the human host will be answered in detail when this emerging procedure is studied in detail (which can be aided by adequate funding and government support) [67]. In the future, these studies will also open our eyes to the benefits MET has over FMT, and whether there are risks associated with the MET procedure. This information will give the medical community a holistic idea about the merits and demerits of the MET procedure, and will allow the medical practitioners (and patients) to make an informed decision on whether to use MET or stick to FMT or antibiotic administration (or a combination of either two of the three options, or combination of the three options). It will also be interesting to find out whether the MET procedure will be effective in the treatment of extra-intestinal diseases in the nearest future [67].

For the advancement of personalized medicine, another prospect is the use of antimicrobial peptides and/or nucleic acid-based methods to selectively kill pathogenic microorganisms in the gut without compromising the structure or function of the gut microbiota (a prominent demerit of antibiotics usage) [69]. Probiotic strains and the gut microbiota have also been thought of as reliable sources of new antimicrobial peptides and antimicrobials, such as bacteriocins [70]. This is because of the complex interaction between the microbial community and its host, especially in the production of metabolites that are active against a narrow spectrum and a broad spectrum of invasive pathogens. Nanotechnological and genetic engineering approaches could widen the precision and spectrum of activity of bacteriocins in future, making them the next generation of antimicrobials [71]. If these products can be utilized, they can effectively guard against antimicrobial resistance (in addition to the maintenance of gut microbial homeostasis) and can serve as therapeutic alternatives in the treatment of inflammatory bowel diseases, irritable bowel syndrome, colorectal cancer, and extra-intestinal diseases such as diabetes. Scientists believe that probiotics will replace antibiotics as drugs vetted by the FDA and European regulatory bodies in the nearest future. This laudable goal is dependent on the correct identification of probiotic strains (with the aid of next-generation sequencing technologies), the palatability of these strains to the sensory organ, validated storage and transport of intact cells to the gut (via microencapsulation approaches, or functional foods, and the fulfillment of all requirements and validation of all necessary stages for its approval as a new drug [72].

There is also a proposal that gut microbes can be genetically engineered so that they possess characteristics that detect what food is present in the gut, monitor inflammation, detect and fight against gastrointestinal pathogens thereby reducing reliance on antibiotics, and exert extra-intestinal effects such as the regulation of behavior and mood and treatment of cancer [73]. Genetically engineered microbes have been reported to be effective against *Vibrio cholerae* in mice especially when this pathogen was ingested 8 hours after the administration of the genetically engineered microbe [74]. There are still many ongoing trials seeking to manipulate and monitor the activities of genetically-engineered microbes in the gut, albeit in animal models. These microbes have to be tested for their safety and their ability to be fit enough to endure gastrointestinal conditions (stomach acid and bile) and successfully colonize the host's gut [75]. There is also the fear about the effect of horizontal recombinant gene transfer on the natural gut commensals. Although microbiome engineering is challenging, it is expected that this strategy will be less expensive and more effective than the traditional methods of gastrointestinal and other extra-intestinal disease control if achieved [76]. The major goal of genetic manipulation of gut microbes is to improve the health of humans.

## 8. Conclusions

One of the most effective ways to reduce the abundance of multi-drug resistant pathogens is with the use of beneficial microorganisms and/or their metabolites, analogous to the effective environmentally-friendly biological method of eliminating stubborn pests in farmlands by agriculturalists. The benefits of the gut microbiota are being constantly unraveled as advanced next-generation sequencing techniques arise. The field of microbio-therapeutics is steadily growing. Harnessing the potentials of these microbes is paramount to making the world a healthier and better place to live.

## Conflict of interest

The authors declare that there is no conflict of interest.

## Author details

Ayorinde O. Afolayan, Adewale Adetoye and Funmilola A. Ayeni*

*Address all correspondence to: funmiyeni@yahoo.co.uk

Department of Pharmaceutical Microbiology, Faculty of Pharmacy, University of Ibadan, Ibadan, Nigeria

## References

[1] Gilbert JA, Neufeld JD. Life in a world without microbes. PLoS Biology. 2014;**12**(12): e1002020. DOI: 10.1371/journal.pbio.1002020

[2] Nagpal R, Kumar A, Arora S. In vitro probiotic potential of lactobacilli isolated from indigenous fermented milk products. International Journal of Probiotics and Prebiotics. 2010;**5**(2):105-112. Available from: http://www.nchpjournals.com/manuscript/uploads/article_818.pdf

[3] Davies J, Davies D. Origins and evolution of antibiotic resistance. Microbiology and Molecular Biology Reviews. 2010 Sep;**74**(3):417-433. Available from: http://www.ncbi.nlm.nih.gov/pubmed/20805405

[4] Center for Disease Control and Prevention. Section 3: Current antibiotic resistance threats in the United States, by microorganism. In: Antibiotic Resistance Threats in the United States [Internet]. Atlanta, USA: Center for Disease Control and Prevention; 2013. pp. 53-54. Available from: https://www.cdc.gov/drugresistance/threat-report-2013/pdf/ar-threats-2013-1

[5] FAO of the UN, WHO. Joint FAO/WHO working group report on drafting guidelines for the evaluation of probiotics in food guidelines for the evaluation of probiotics in food report of a joint FAO/WHO working group on drafting guidelines for the evaluation of probiotics in food [Internet]. 2002. Available from: http://www.who.int/foodsafety/fs_management/en/probiotic_guidelines.pdf

[6] Nissle A. Explanations of the significance of colonic dysbacteria & the mechanism of action of *E. coli* therapy (mutaflor). Medizinische. 1959;**4**(21):1017-1022. Available from: http://www.ncbi.nlm.nih.gov/pubmed/13673841

[7] Czerucka D, Piche T, Rampal P. Yeast as probiotics—*Saccharomyces boulardii*. Alimentary Pharmacology & Therapeutics. 2007;**26**(6):767-778

[8] Ayeni FA, Adeniyi BA, Ogunbanwo ST, Tabasco R, Paarup T, Peláez C, et al. Inhibition of uropathogens by lactic acid bacteria isolated from dairy foods and cow's intestine in western Nigeria. Archives of Microbiology. 2009;**191**(8):639-648. Available from: http://link.springer.com/10.1007/s00203-009-0492-9

[9] Ayeni FA, Sánchez B, Adeniyi BA, de los Reyes-Gavilán CG, Margolles A, Ruas-Madiedo P. Evaluation of the functional potential of Weissella and *Lactobacillus* isolates obtained from Nigerian traditional fermented foods and cow's intestine. International Journal of

Food Microbiology. 2011;**147**(2):97-104. Available from: http://www.ncbi.nlm.nih.gov/pubmed/21482440

[10] Toshimitsu T, Ozaki S, Mochizuki J, Furuichi K, Asami Y. Effects of *Lactobacillus plantarum* strain OLL2712 culture conditions on the anti-inflammatory activities for murine immune cells and obese and type 2 diabetic mice. Applied Environmental Microbiology. 2017 Apr 1;**83**(7):e03001-e03016. Available from: http://www.ncbi.nlm.nih.gov/pubmed/28087537

[11] Fonseca W, Lucey K, Jang S, Fujimura KE, Rasky A, Ting H-A, et al. *Lactobacillus johnsonii* supplementation attenuates respiratory viral infection via metabolic reprogramming and immune cell modulation. Mucosal Immunology. 2017 Nov 15;**10**(6):1569-1580. Available from: http://www.ncbi.nlm.nih.gov/pubmed/28295020

[12] Shonyela SM, Wang G, Yang W, Yang G, Wang CF. New progress regarding the use of lactic acid bacteria as live delivery vectors, treatment of diseases and induction of immune responses in different host species focusing on *Lactobacillus* species. [cited 2018 Jun 2]. Available from: https://www.omicsonline.org/open-access/new-progress-regarding-the-use-of-lactic-acid-bacteria-as-live-deliveryvectors-treatment-of-diseases-and-induction-of-immune-respo-2329-8901-1000187.pdf

[13] Bharwani A, Mian MF, Surette MG, Bienenstock J, Forsythe P. Oral treatment with *Lactobacillus rhamnosus* attenuates behavioural deficits and immune changes in chronic social stress. BMC Medicine. 2017 Dec 11;**15**(1):7. Available from: http://www.ncbi.nlm.nih.gov/pubmed/28073366

[14] Wang H, Lee I-S, Braun C, Enck P. Effect of probiotics on central nervous system functions in animals and humans: A systematic review. Journal of Neurogastroenterology and Motility. 2016;**22**(4):589-605. Available from: http://www.ncbi.nlm.nih.gov/pubmed/27413138

[15] O'Hara AM, Shanahan F. Mechanisms of action of probiotics in intestinal diseases. The Scientific World Journal. 2007 Jan 10;**7**:31-46. Available from: http://www.ncbi.nlm.nih.gov/pubmed/17221140

[16] Kruis W, Fric P, Pokrotnieks J, Lukás M, Fixa B, Kascák M, et al. Maintaining remission of ulcerative colitis with the probiotic *Escherichia coli* Nissle 1917 is as effective as with standard mesalazine. Gut. 2004 Nov 1;**53**(11):1617-1623. Available from: http://www.ncbi.nlm.nih.gov/pubmed/15479682

[17] Ouwehand AC, Forssten S, Hibberd AA, Lyra A, Stahl B. Probiotic approach to prevent antibiotic resistance. Annals of Medicine. 2016;**48**(4):246-255. Available from: https://www.tandfonline.com/doi/full/10.3109/07853890.2016.1161232

[18] Shewale RN, Sawale PD, Khedkar C, Singh A, Sawale PD. Selection criteria for probiotics: A review. International Journal of Probiotics and Prebiotics. 2014;**9**(12):17-22. Available from: https://pdfs.semanticscholar.org/5725/3cf371060b670a3c6e744202a62bc2a3dd99.pdf?_ga=2.76295957.1223746562.1527917940-1231800144.1522095415

[19] Modzelewska-Kapituła M, Kłębukowska L, Kazimierz Kornacki WŁ. Characterization of probiotic properties of *Lactobacillus* strains. Polish Journal of Natural Science. 2008;**23**(2): 366-373. Available from: https://www.researchgate.net/profile/Irena_Brzozowska/publication/251007015_Nadmiary_I_Niedobory_Opadow_W_Polsce_Polnocno-Wschodniej/links/5672b52a08aedbbb3f9f51a0.pdf#page=103

[20] Government of Canada, Health Canada, Health Products and Food Branch NHPD. Ingredient Search. 2004. Available from: http://webprod.hc-sc.gc.ca/nhpid-bdipsn/atReq.do?atid=probio

[21] FDA. Microorganisms & Microbial-Derived Ingredients Used in Food (Partial List). Food And Drug Administration, Center for Food Safety and Applied Nutrition; 2015. Available from: https://www.fda.gov/Food/IngredientsPackagingLabeling/GRAS/MicroorganismsMicrobialDerivedIngredients/default.htm

[22] WGO. World Gastroenterology Organization Global Guidelines on Probiotics and Prebiotics. February 2017

[23] Figueroa-González I, Quijano G, Ramírez G, Cruz-Guerrero A. Probiotics and prebiotics—Perspectives and challenges. Journal of the Science of Food and Agriculture. 2011;**91**(8):1341-1348

[24] Saranraj P, M A N, Sivasakthivelan P. Lactic acid bacteria and its antimicrobial properties: A review. International Journal of Pharmaceutical and Biological Science Archive. 2013;**4**(6):1124-1133

[25] Ricke S. Perspectives on the use of organic acids and short chain fatty acids as antimicrobials. Poultry Science. 2003 Apr 1;**82**(4):632-639. Available from: http://www.ncbi.nlm.nih.gov/pubmed/12710485

[26] Gillor O, Etzion A, Riley MA. The dual role of bacteriocins as anti- and probiotics. Applied Microbiology and Biotechnology. 2008;**81**(4):591-606

[27] Zacharof MP, Lovitt RW. Bacteriocins produced by lactic acid bacteria a review article. APCBEE Procedia. 2012 Jan 1;**2**:50-56. Available from: https://www.sciencedirect.com/science/article/pii/S2212670812000814

[28] Chen H, Hoover DG. Bacteriocins and their food applications. Comprehensive Reviews in Food Science and Food Safety. 2003;**2**(3):82-100. Available from: http://doi.wiley.com/10.1111/j.1541-4337.2003.tb00016.x

[29] Perez RH, Zendo T, Sonomoto K. Novel bacteriocins from lactic acid bacteria (LAB): Various structures and applications. Microbial Cell Factories. 2014;**13**:S3

[30] Deegan LH, Cotter PD, Ross P. Bacteriocins: Biological tools for bio-preservation and shelf-life extension. International Dairy Journal. 2006;**16**(9):1058-1071. Available from: https://www.sciencedirect.com/science/article/pii/S0958694605002827

[31] Liévin-Le Moal V, Servin AL. Anti-infective activities of *Lactobacillus* strains in the human intestinal microbiota: From probiotics to gastrointestinal anti-infectious biotherapeutic

agents. Clinical Microbiology Reviews. 2014 Apr;**27**(2):167-199. Available from: http://www.ncbi.nlm.nih.gov/pubmed/24696432

[32] Gordon DM, O'Brien CL. Bacteriocin diversity and the frequency of multiple bacteriocin production in *Escherichia coli*. Microbiology. 2006;**152**(11):3239-3244. Available from: http://www.ncbi.nlm.nih.gov/pubmed/17074895

[33] Kerac M, Bunn J, Seal A, Thindwa M, Tomkins A, Sadler K, et al. Probiotics and prebiotics for severe acute malnutrition (PRONUT study): A double-blind efficacy randomised controlled trial in Malawi. Lancet. 2009 Jul 11;**374**(9684):136-144. Available from: http://www.ncbi.nlm.nih.gov/pubmed/19595348

[34] de Vrese M, Marteau PR. Probiotics and prebiotics: Effects on diarrhea. The Journal of Nutrition. 2007 Mar 1;**137**(3):803S-811S. Available from: https://academic.oup.com/jn/article/137/3/803S/4664760

[35] Pandey KR, Naik SR, Vakil BV. Probiotics, prebiotics and synbiotics- a review. Journal of Food Science and Technology. 2015 Dec;**52**(12):7577-7587. Available from: http://www.ncbi.nlm.nih.gov/pubmed/26604335

[36] Adeniyi BA, Adetoye A, Ayeni FA. Antibacterial activities of lactic acid bacteria isolated from cow faeces against potential enteric pathogens. African Health Sciences. 2015 Sep;**15**(3):888-895. Available from: http://www.ncbi.nlm.nih.gov/pubmed/26957978

[37] Afolayan AO, Ayeni FA, Ruppitsch W. Antagonistic and quantitative assessment of indigenous lactic acid bacteria in different varieties of ogi against gastrointestinal pathogens. The Pan African Medical Journal. 2017;**27**(22):eCollections 2017

[38] Niyogi SK. Shigellosis. Journal of Microbiology. 2005 Apr;**43**(2):133-143. Available from: http://www.ncbi.nlm.nih.gov/pubmed/15880088

[39] Mirnejad R, Vahdati AR, Rashidiani J, Erfani M, Piranfar V. The antimicrobial effect of *Lactobacillus casei* culture supernatant against multiple drug resistant clinical isolates of *Shigella sonnei* and *Shigella flexneri* in vitro. Iranian Red Crescent Medical Journal. 2013 Feb;**15**(2):122-126. Available from: http://www.ncbi.nlm.nih.gov/pubmed/23682323

[40] Afolayan AO, Ayeni FA. Antagonistic effects of three lactic acid bacterial strains isolated from Nigerian indigenous fermented ogi on *E. coli* EKT004 in co-culture. Acta Alimentaria. 2017;**46**(1):1-8

[41] Ayeni AO, Ruppitsch W, Ayeni FA. Characterization of bacteria in Nigerian yogurt as promising alternative to antibiotics in gastrointestinal infections. Journal of Dietary Supplements. 2018 Mar 14:1-11. Available from: https://www.tandfonline.com/doi/full/10.1080/19390211.2018.1440684

[42] Majowicz SE, Musto J, Scallan E, Angulo FJ, Kirk M, O'Brien SJ, et al. The global burden of nontyphoidal *Salmonella* gastroenteritis. Clinical Infectious Diseases. 2010 Mar 15;**50**(6):882-889. Available from: http://www.ncbi.nlm.nih.gov/pubmed/20158401

[43] Abdel-Daim A, Hassouna N, Hafez M, Ashor MSA, Aboulwafa MM. Antagonistic activity of *Lactobacillus* isolates against *Salmonella typhi In Vitro*. BioMed Research International. 2013;**2013**:1-12. Available from: http://www.ncbi.nlm.nih.gov/pubmed/24191248

[44] Casey PG, Gardiner GE, Casey G, Bradshaw B, Lawlor PG, Lynch PB, et al. A five-strain probiotic combination reduces pathogen shedding and alleviates disease signs in pigs challenged with *Salmonella enterica* Serovar Typhimurium. Applied and Environmental Microbiology. 2007 Mar 15;**73**(6):1858-1863. Available from: http://www.ncbi.nlm.nih.gov/pubmed/17261517

[45] Alebiosu KM, Adetoye A, Ayeni F. Antimicrobial activities of lactic acid bacteria against *Pseudomonas aeruginosa, Providencia vermicola, Alcaligenes faecalis* and methicillin resistant *S. aureus*. West African Journal of Pharmacy. 2017;**28**(2):132-142

[46] Guay DRP. Contemporary management of uncomplicated urinary tract infections. Drugs. 2008;**68**(9):1169-1205. Available from: http://link.springer.com/10.2165/00003495-200868090-00002

[47] Reid G, Bruce AW. Probiotics to prevent urinary tract infections: The rationale and evidence. World Journal of Urology. 2006 Feb;**24**(1):28-32. Available from: http://www.ncbi.nlm.nih.gov/pubmed/16389539

[48] Adeniyi BA, Ayeni FA, Ogunbanwo ST. Antagonistic activities of lactic acid bacteria isolated from Nigerian fermented dairy food against organisms implicated in urinary tract infection. Biotechnology (Faisalabad). 2006 Feb 1;**5**(2):183-188. Available from: http://www.scialert.net/abstract/?doi=biotech.2006.183.188

[49] Ayeni F, Adeniyi B. Antimicrobial potentials of lactic acid bacteria isolated from a Nigerian menstruating woman. TAF Preventive Medicine Bulletin. 2013;**12**(3):283. Available from: http://www.scopemed.org/fulltextpdf.php?mno=21566

[50] Graver MA, Wade JJ. The role of acidification in the inhibition of *Neisseria gonorrhoeae* by vaginal lactobacilli during anaerobic growth. Annals of Clinical Microbiology and Antimicrobials. 2011;**10**(1):8. Available from: http://www.ncbi.nlm.nih.gov/pubmed/21329492

[51] Bamidele A, Adeniyi B, Ogunbanwo S, Smith S, Omonigbehin E. Antibacterial activities of lactic acid bacteria isolated from selected vegetables grown in Nigeria: A preliminary report. Sierra Leone Journal of Biomedical Research. 2018;**3**(3):128-132. Available from: https://www.ajol.info/index.php/sljbr/article/view/74040

[52] Awaad AS, AL-Mudhayyif HA, Al-Othman MR, Zain ME, El-Meligy RM. Amhezole, a novel fungal secondary metabolite from *Aspergillus terreus* for treatment of microbial mouth infection. Phytherapy Research. 2017 Mar;**31**(3):395-402. Available from: http://www.ncbi.nlm.nih.gov/pubmed/28083890

[53] Yang Y, Song H, Wang L, Dong W, Yang Z, Yuan P, et al. Antiviral effects of a probiotic metabolic products against transmissible gastroenteritis coronavirus. Journal of Probiotics and Health. 2017;**5**(3):1-6. Available from: https://www.omicsonline.org/open-access/antiviral-effects-of-a-probiotic-metabolic-products-against-transmissible-gastroenteritis-coronavirus-2329-8901-1000184.php?aid=94025

[54] Guarino A, Guandalini S, Lo Vecchio A. Probiotics for prevention and treatment of diarrhea. Journal of Clinical Gastroenterology. 2015;**49**:S37-S45. Available from: http://www.ncbi.nlm.nih.gov/pubmed/26447963

[55] Belkaid Y, Hand TW. Role of the microbiota in immunity and inflammation. Cell. 2014 Mar 27;**157**(1):121-141. Available from: http://www.cell.com/abstract/S0092-8674(14)00345-6

[56] Beaud D, Tailliez P, Anba-Mondoloni J. Genetic characterization of the beta-glucuronidase enzyme from a human intestinal bacterium, *Ruminococcus gnavus*. Microbiology. 2005 Jul 1;**151**(7):2323-2330. Available from: http://www.ncbi.nlm.nih.gov/pubmed/16000722

[57] Kashyap PC, Chia N, Nelson H, Segal E, Elinav E. Microbiome at the frontier of personalized medicine. Mayo Clinic Proceedings. 2017 Dec 1;**92**(12):1855-1864. Available from: https://www.sciencedirect.com/science/article/pii/S0025619617307322

[58] Schnorr SL, Candela M, Rampelli S, Centanni M, Consolandi C, Basaglia G, et al. Gut microbiome of the Hadza hunter-gatherers. Nature Communications. 2014 Apr 15;**5**:3654. Available from: http://www.nature.com/doifinder/10.1038/ncomms4654

[59] Forbes JD, Van Domselaar G, Bernstein CN. The gut microbiota in immune-mediated inflammatory diseases. Frontiers in Microbiology. 2016;**7**:1081. Available from: http://www.ncbi.nlm.nih.gov/pubmed/27462309

[60] Biagi E, Nylund L, Candela M, Ostan R, Bucci L, Pini E, et al. Through ageing, and beyond: Gut microbiota and inflammatory status in seniors and centenarians. PLoS One. 2010 May 17;**5**(5):e10667. Available from: http://dx.plos.org/10.1371/journal.pone.0010667

[61] Kaufmann SHE. Immunology's foundation: The 100-year anniversary of the Nobel prize to Paul Ehrlich and Elie Metchnikoff. Nature Immunology. 2008 Jul 1;**9**(7):705-712. Available from: http://www.ncbi.nlm.nih.gov/pubmed/18563076

[62] Téllez G, Lauková A, Latorre JD, Hernandez-Velasco X, Hargis BM, Callaway T. Food-producing animals and their health in relation to human health. Microbial Ecology in Health and Disease. 2015;**26**:25876. Available from: http://www.ncbi.nlm.nih.gov/pubmed/25651994

[63] Imperial ICVJ, Ibana JA. Addressing the antibiotic resistance problem with probiotics: Reducing the risk of its double-edged sword effect. Frontiers in Microbiology. 2016;**7**:1983. Available from: http://www.ncbi.nlm.nih.gov/pubmed/28018315

[64] Aroniadis OC, Brandt LJ. Fecal microbiota transplantation. Current Opinion in Gastroenterology. 2013 Jan;**29**(1):79-84. Available from: http://content.wkhealth.com/linkback/openurl?sid=WKPTLP:landingpage&an=00001574-201301000-00014

[65] Terveer EM, van Beurden YH, Goorhuis A, Seegers JFML, Bauer MP, van Nood E, et al. How to: Establish and run a stool bank. Clinical Microbiology and Infection. 2017 Dec 1;**23**(12):924-930. Available from: https://www.sciencedirect.com/science/article/pii/S1198743X17302756

[66] Mistroff J, Iv M, Guzzardo G, Iii M, Salem A, Cornelious M, et al. Cultured media containing bacterial flora could be a better alternative to fecal transplantation in treating recurrent *Clostridium difficile* colitis. Journal of Clinical & Experimental Immunology. 2016;**1**(4). Available from: http://www.opastonline.com/wp-content/uploads/2017/01/

cultured-media-containing-bacterial-flora-could-be-a-better-alternative-to-fecal-transplantation-in-treating-recurrent-clostridium-difficile-colitis-jcei-16-008.pdf

[67] Allen-Vercoe E, Petrof EO. Using bugs as drugs: Microbial ecosystem therapeutics. Canada Communicable Disease Report. 2015;**45**(Suppl 5):3-6. Available from: http://www.ncbi.nlm.nih.gov/pubmed/29770104

[68] Petrof EO, Gloor GB, Vanner SJ, Weese SJ, Carter D, Daigneault MC, et al. Stool substitute transplant therapy for the eradication of *Clostridium difficile* infection: RePOOPulating the gut. Microbiome. 2013;**1**(1):3. Available from: http://www.ncbi.nlm.nih.gov/pubmed/24467987

[69] de la Fuente-Nunez C, Torres MD, Mojica FJ, Lu TK. Next-generation precision antimicrobials: Towards personalized treatment of infectious diseases. Current Opinion in Microbiology. 2017;**37**:95-102. Available from: DOI: 10.1016/j.mib.2017.05.014

[70] Garcia-Gutierrez E, Mayer MJ, Cotter PD, Narbad A. Gut microbiota as a source of novel antimicrobials. Gut Microbes. 2018:1-21. [Epub ahead of print]. Available from: https://www.tandfonline.com/doi/full/10.1080/19490976.2018.1455790

[71] Gillor O, Nigro LM, Riley M. Genetically engineered bacteriocins and their potential as the next generation of antimicrobials. Current Pharmaceutical Design. 2005;**11**:1067-1075

[72] FDA. Code of Federal Regulations Title 21. Vol. 3. 2016. Available from: https://www.accessdata.fda.gov/scripts/cdrh/cfdocs/cfcfr/CFRSearch.cfm?CFRPart=312&showFR=1&subpartNode=21:5.0.1.1.3.2

[73] Sonnenburg JL. Microbiome engineering. Nature. 2015;**518**(7540):S10. Available from: http://www.nature.com/articles/518S10a

[74] Duan F, March JC. Engineered bacterial communication prevents Vibrio cholerae virulence in an infant mouse model. Proceedings of the National Academy of the Sciences of the United States of America. 2010;**107**(25):11260-11264. Available from: http://www.ncbi.nlm.nih.gov/pubmed/20534565

[75] Lu TK, Mimee M, Citorik RJ, Pepper K. Engineering the microbiome for human health applications. In: The Chemistry of Microbiomes: Proceedings of a Seminar Series. Washington, DC: National Academies Press; 2017. Available from: https://www.nap.edu/catalog/24751

[76] Landry BP, Tabor JJ. Engineering diagnostic and therapeutic gut bacteria. Microbiology Spectrum. 2017;**5**(5). Available from: http://www.ncbi.nlm.nih.gov/pubmed/29052539